Integrative Framing Analysis

While there is a plethora of visual communication and media framing books, there is a paucity of research that combines both textual and visual framing approaches. Viorela Dan's book is well positioned to fill this important scholarly gap in the area of framing analysis. Building on theoretical and methodological strengths of existing framing studies, the book offers a clear and comprehensive overview of what has been done in this area to date and where we need to go from here. The book will provide an invaluable resource for graduate-level seminars in Media Framing, Health Communication, Mass Communication Theory, Research Methods, and International Communication.

—Daniela V. Dimitrova, Iowa State University, USA

Much of framing scholarship focuses exclusively on the analysis either of words or of visuals. This book addresses this gap by proposing an approach to the analysis of verbal frames, visual frames, and the interplay between them: an integrative framing analysis. This approach is demonstrated through a study investigating the way words and visuals are used to frame people living with HIV/AIDS in various communication contexts: the news, public service announcements, and special interest publications. This application of integrative framing analysis reveals differences between verbal frames and visual frames in the same messages, underscoring the importance of looking at these frames together.

Viorela Dan (Dr. phil. 2016, Free University of Berlin) is a Research Associate at the Institute for Media and Communication Studies of the Free University of Berlin, Germany. She received the Promising Professor Award in 2013 (third place, AEJMC) and the Highly Commended Paper Award in 2011 (Elsevier). Some of her previous publications include articles in the *International Journal of Press/Politics* and *Journal of Communication Management.*

Routledge Research in Communication Studies

1 **Populist Political Communication in Europe**
Edited by Toril Aalberg, Frank Esser, Carsten Reinemann, Jesper Strömbäck, and Claes H. de Vreese

2 **Setting Agendas in Cultural Markets**
Organizations, Creators, Experiences
Philemon Bantimaroudis

3 **Communication, Advocacy, and Work/Family Balance**
Jenny Dixon

4 **Integrative Framing Analysis**
Framing Health through Words and Visuals
Viorela Dan

Integrative Framing Analysis

Framing Health through Words and Visuals

Viorela Dan

Routledge
Taylor & Francis Group
NEW YORK AND LONDON

First published 2018 by Routledge

2 Park Square, Milton Park, Abingdon, Oxfordshire OX14 4RN
52 Vanderbilt Avenue, New York, NY 10017

Routledge is an imprint of the Taylor & Francis Group, an informa business

First issued in paperback 2019

An earlier version of this book served as the author's doctoral dissertation submitted in partial fulfillment of the requirements for the degree of Dr. phil. to the Department of Political and Social Sciences of the Freie Universität Berlin in Berlin, Germany in 2016. Juliana Raupp, Freie Universität Berlin and Renita Coleman, University of Texas at Austin served as advisers and co-chairs of the doctoral committee.

Library of Congress Cataloging-in-Publication Data
CIP data has been applied for.

ISBN: 978-1-138-04636-8 (hbk)
ISBN: 978-0-367-88908-1 (pbk)

DOI: 10.4324/9781315171456

Typeset in Sabon
by codeMantra

To my wonderful *Doktormüttern*,
Juliana Raupp, Freie Universität Berlin and
Renita Coleman, University of Texas at Austin,
with my deepest gratitude

Contents

List of Figures and Tables

Figures

Tables

List of Abbreviations

χ^2	Approximate Chi-Square
AIDS	Acquired Immunodeficiency Syndrome
amfAR	The American Foundation for AIDS Research
CDC	Centers for Disease Control and Prevention
CR_{Frames}	Verbal-Visual Frame Congruence Ratio
DCT	Dual Coding Theory
DTCA	Direct-to-Consumer Pharmaceutical Advertising for Prescription Drugs
ELM	Elaboration Likelihood Model
HIV	Human Immunodeficiency Virus[1]
HSM	Heuristic Systematic Model
JFCoI	Janis Fadner Coefficient of Imbalance
KFF	The Henry J. Kaiser Family Foundation
LCM	Limited Capacity Model
LGBT	Lesbian, Gay, Bisexual, and Transgender
MD	Mean Difference
N/A	Not Applicable
$Pairs_{=}$	Number of Frame Pairs
Pew	The Pew Research Center
PLWHA	Person/People Living with HIV or AIDS
PSA/s	Public Service Announcement/s
PSE	Picture Superiority Effect
SIP/s	Special-Interest/ Niche Publication/s
$\Sigma_{Visual\ Frames}$	Total Number of Visual Frames

1 According to the CDC, an infection with HIV deteriorates one's immune system by attacking CD4 cells (also known as T cells). One's body can then no longer efficiently deter disease and infection, making individuals more susceptible to rare cancers and opportunistic infections. Such symptoms indicate that person has reached the third and last stage of disease, known as AIDS (Centers for Disease Control and Prevention, 2013b).

1 Introduction

Traditionally, social science has been an "obstinately verbal" field (Fyfe & Law, 1988, p. 4) in which scholars have shown a clear preference for the analysis of words over visuals. Visuals were considered "intellectual[ly] lightweight" (Grabe & Bucy, 2009, p. 67), "pandering to [the] low tastes" (Becker, 1995, p. 9) of "the subhuman, the savage, the 'dumb' animal, the child, the woman *[sic]*, the masses" (Mitchell, 1994, p. 24; Postman, 1986). Other reasons for dismissing visuals included their ubiquity in tabloids and their capacity to stir emotions and to manipulate (impressionable) audiences (see Bergstroem, 2008; Habermas, 1989).

Given this pervasive "word bias"[1] (Grabe & Bucy, 2009, p. 6), researchers who shut their eyes to visuals did not have to justify their position for many years. This changed because of the devotion of a few researchers—particularly Doris Graber (1980, 1986, 1987, 1988)—to visual analyses. For these scholars, visuals' omnipresence, their exploitation for strategic purposes, and their accessibility to those less educated made them more interesting for research, not less (see also Grabe & Bucy, 2009).

Acknowledging this has led to a growing interest in "all things visual" (Hughes, 2012, p. xxix). This interest is clear in the discipline-wide praise of studies focusing on the visual channel of communication. *Image bite politics*—Grabe and Bucy's 2009 monograph—was surely one of the landmark publications of recent years to strengthen the case for studying visuals. Even so, scholars must acknowledge that visual-only studies, just like verbal-only studies, are incomplete (see Coleman, 2010; Graber, 1987). Audiences are not exposed to *either* the verbal *or* the visual components of a message but rather to *both* words *and* visuals. Thus, at a time when the hurdles associated with researching visuals have been progressively reduced, our discipline must move toward "integrative work" (Coleman, 2010, p. 235) that analyzes both words and visuals. In this book, I investigate the feasibility of integrative analyses by focusing on framing theory.

Various definitions of frames and framing circulate in the academe (see Coleman, 2010; Entman, 1993; Entman, Matthes, & Pellicano, 2008; Reese, 2001). In my understanding, frames are rather enduring verbal or

DOI: 10.4324/9781315171456-1

visual interpretations of issues or people. Frames seem natural to those whose ideas, norms, or values they reference. They organize social reality, simplifying complex matters by emphasizing certain aspects and disregarding others. Full-fledged frames define a state of affairs as problematic, suggest moral evaluations, identify causes, and propose ways to alleviate the problem. The treatment recommendations, especially, give frames their functional character by making certain policies, attitudes, or behaviors seem like the natural response to the problem. Visuals can convey frames by themselves, and these frames can be similar to or different from those articulated verbally in the same message. Visual frames fulfill the four framing functions outlined by Entman (1993) through the content of the visual and, possibly, in less obvious ways (e.g., through variations in nonverbal behavior, camera angles, and camera distances). Frames are available in culture, in communication (written and spoken words; still and moving images), and in people's minds. Framing is the act of developing and promoting frames. In this way, frames pertain to issues or people. The latter group, frames about people, is known as "character frames." Grabe and Bucy (2009) introduced the term "character frames" in reference to politicians running for office. Through character frames, some aspects of people's personalities and lives are selected and highlighted in verbal or visual communication, while others are disregarded or downplayed. Aspects may be chosen for emphasis to explain why a certain individual got into the state described or portrayed, to suggest a moral evaluation, or to propose ways to deal with that individual's current state. Character frames organize social reality and make certain policies, attitudes, or behaviors seem like the natural response to the problem described or portrayed. Investigating character frames is worthwhile as the way in which journalists and other actors communicate about those most directly affected by an issue can impact audiences' perception of the issue as a whole more than baseline statistics.

Coleman's (2010) call for integrative framing analyses set in motion the train of thought for this book. The point of departure for my investigation into their feasibility was my expectation that they would be twice as laborious as verbal-only or visual-only studies. Nonetheless, I expected the effort to be manageable—given the wide availability of methodological advice on both verbal and visual framing analyses (e.g., Coleman, 2010; David, Atun, Fille, & Monterola, 2011; Matthes & Kohring, 2008; Messaris & Abraham, 2001; Tankard, 2001; Van Gorp, 2010)—and, more important, worth the effort. But it soon became evident that mastering the body of knowledge associated with verbal and visual framing analyses, respectively, was only the first step in coming to grips with integrative framing analyses. Many questions about how words and visuals can relate to each other unfolded in the process. This reinforced my belief that the lack of precise, hands-on, methodological guidance on the integration of words and visuals was responsible for the small number of integrative framing analyses to date. In this book, I hope to blaze the trail for those considering embarking on such studies themselves. I propose a step-by-step approach to integrative framing analysis and implement it in an empirical study to demonstrate that it is feasible and effective.

The remainder of this book is divided into six chapters. Chapter 2 testifies to the need for integrative framing analyses by offering three arguments based on previous studies. One argument is that most messages consist of words and visuals (Kress, 2010) and that, on many occasions, visuals are the dominant element of such messages. A second line of reasoning draws on a vast body of experimental research that strongly suggested that visuals were awarded more attention and preferential processing than words (e.g., Holsanova, Rahm, & Holmqvist, 2006; Knobloch, Hastall, Zillmann, & Callison, 2003; Zillmann, Knobloch, & Yu, 2001). Finally, I review another corpus of studies investigating memory and recall for information conveyed verbally and/or visually. Here, it becomes apparent that messages conveyed visually are better at attracting attention than words are (e.g., Bucher & Schumacher, 2006; Donsbach, 1991; Garcia & Stark, 1991). But even in the unlikely event that audiences pay equal attention to words and visuals in a given message, there is no reason to focus solely on the verbal component of that message. As discussed in Chapter 2 in depth, when words and visuals do not convey the same information, which is frequently the case, audiences are much more likely to retain the information conveyed through visuals than through words (e.g., Bucy & Newhagen, 1999; Grimes, 1991; Lang, 1995).

In Chapter 3, I describe the difficulties associated with integrative framing analyses. I argue that a first challenge is posed by the wide array of approaches to verbal framing analyses and visual framing analyses, respectively (Coleman, 2010; Matthes & Kohring, 2008; Rodriguez & Dimitrova, 2011). The difficulty lies in deciding which of the approaches available makes the most sense for addressing one's particular research questions and hypotheses. As discussed in depth in this chapter, this decision can be particularly troublesome for visual framing, given the lack of clarity concerning the way to extract meaning from visuals. Scholars differ greatly in this regard. Drawing on the "methodological trail of breadcrumbs" provided by Coleman (2010) with the intention "to help framing scholars feel less lost in the visual forest" (p. 235); on Grabe and Bucy's (2009) empirical study on visual character frames; and on Rodriguez and Dimitrova's (2011) systematization of visual framing studies, and assisted by insights from Geise, Lobinger, and Brantner (2013), this chapter presents the five different foci chosen by framing scholars who include visuals in their analyses. A detailed review reveals that—regardless of their focus on the verbal or the visual modality—some approaches have more weaknesses than others, but they resonate with researchers nonetheless. Thus, I pose that scholars' choice of one approach or the other depends not just on an evaluation of strengths and weaknesses, but also on its suitability for answering one's research questions, on one's understanding of frames, one's methodological preferences, cost-benefit calculations, and, finally, on efforts toward methodological triangulation.

Then, after the presentation of approaches to verbal and visual framing analyses when conducted individually, the approaches to integrative framing analyses identified in previous studies are reviewed. Here, I argue that one of the two approaches currently circulating in the literature has a clear advantage over the other. Specifically, in keeping with the literature reviewed in Chapter 2, I suggest that collecting data separately from words and visuals is much more valuable than attempting to do this simultaneously. Nonetheless, with this field of research still in its infancy, it becomes apparent that the sequence of steps to be followed in such analyses is far from clear. The question of precisely how to conduct integrative analyses when collecting data separately from words and visuals arises at the end of Chapter 3. This question is addressed in Chapter 5.

But first, in Chapter 4, I turn to the factors influencing the acts of selection and emphasis inherent to framing. Why do journalists and other communicators use the frames that they do? Based on previous research on frame building, however scarce, I explain how framing can sometimes occur unconsciously, because of the resonance of certain interpretations with the underlying culture (e.g., Gamson, 1989). I then move to a second explanation, which seems more plausible to me: More often, a communicator's interests and goals motivate that communicator's use of frames (e.g., Hallahan, 2015). I pose that framing analyses are incomplete without an investigation into how frames serve certain interests. Here, I present two lines of research, one attempting to link the prevalence of news sources in a story to news frames (e.g., Dimitrova & Strömbäck, 2012), the other contrasting news frames to frames conveyed by actors external to the media (e.g., Hänggli & Kriesi, 2012). The latter are known as advocacy frames. While previous research identified other factors that impact frame building at the macro-level and meso-level (e.g., Dimitrova & Kostadinova, 2013), they are not at the core of this book.

In Chapter 5, I propose a clearly defined sequence of six steps to be followed, which I demonstrate in the next chapter. They concern the preparation of the material for the analysis, the data collection, and the data analysis. The focus is placed on identifying verbal frames in written text, identifying visual frames in still images, and also on assessing the interplay between them. For the assessment of the interplay, a formula is introduced. It allows the computation of what I call the verbal-visual frame congruence ratio (CR_{Frames}). Applying this formula to the data results in a new interval-level variable that can be used in subsequent analyses.

In Chapter 6, I execute each of these six steps while conducting a study of the frames conveyed through written words and still images about people living with HIV/AIDS (PLWHA) in news, special interest publications (SIPs), and public service announcements (PSAs). This chapter begins with a literature review on the framing of PLWHA and continues with a presentation of hypotheses and research questions. The last sections of the chapter are devoted to the presentation and discussion of the results of the integrative framing analysis of PLWHA. I hope that journalists and communication practitioners can benefit from reading especially this section of the book, as it deals with a variety of factors potentially influencing the framing of PLWHA. Some of the factors whose influence on framing was tested in this study are the communication context (news, SIPs, PSAs), the sourcing practices (news sources, photo sources), the characteristics of the audience (aka community structure; i.e., political views, urban-rural ratio, religiosity, and HIV/AIDS prevalence), and the goals of communication. Finally, several influences on variations in the degree to which verbal frames and visual frames conveyed the same interpretation were tested.

The theoretical and methodological contributions of this book are addressed in Chapter 7. Despite the topic selected for the empirical test of the methodological approach proposed in Chapter 5, this approach can be applied to the study of any topic. I hope that this book can reveal bridges across our discipline as envisioned by Waisbord (2015), tear down the wall between researchers self-identified as either words-people or visuals-people (see Fahmy, Bock, & Wanta, 2014), and lead to an increased number of integrative framing analyses.

Note

1 Hofmann (2008) used, therefore, the harsher term of "verbal snobbery" (p. 270, my translation); see also Gazzaniga (1998).

2 Arguments in Favor of Integrative Framing Analyses

As explained in the Introduction, visual-only studies, just like word-only studies, are necessarily fragmentary (see also Coleman, 2010; Graber, 1987). This chapter presents three arguments in favor of analyzing the contribution of both words and visuals to the framing of people or issues across communication contexts. They concern the ubiquity of multimodal messages and the ways in which visuals outplay words when it comes to attention, processing, memory, and recall.

Multimodal Messages and the Predominance of Visuals

Nowadays, purely verbal messages are typical of little more than radio broadcasting; purely visual messages are equally scarce (see Mitchell, 2005; Müller, 2007). Monomodal messages are artificial by nature. In the words of Kress (2010), multimodal messages (i.e., those in which several modes of communication are used) are "the normal state of human communication" (p. 1).

Multimodality is typical of news accounts (e.g., Kress & van Leeuwen, 1998; Macken-Horarik, 2003; Roosvall, 2016), not just on television (Gunter, 2015; Machin & Niblock, 2006), but also in newspapers (Vobič & Tomanić Trivundža, 2015). Vobič & Tomanić Trivundža (2015) showed how print journalists engaged in a "desperate search for 'any image'," something they termed the "tyranny of the empty frame" (p. 502). Furthermore, messages in magazines and advertising (whether social or commercial) are typically multimodal (Griffin, 2004; Newton, 2001). According to recent studies, visuals became the dominant, and sometimes the only, component of print ads (e.g., Brier, 2009; Gold, Cohen, & Shumate, 2008; Scalvini, 2010)—something that led Lobinger (2012) to the observation that photos are "advertising's darlings" (p. 124). Finally, photos are now a crucial component of magazines (Griffin, 2004; Hull, Smith, & Schmittel, 2015).

More Attention and Preferential Processing for Visuals over Words

In environments glutted with messages, people can only process a small fraction (Findlay & Gilchrist, 2003; Graber & Holyk, 2012). The selection

DOI: 10.4324/9781315171456-2

of the very few stimuli to be further processed is guided by what draws people's attention (Eder, 2002; Hickethier, 2002; Holmqvist, Holsanova, Barthelson, & Lundqvist, 2003; Liu, 2005; Stark Adam, Edmonds, & Quinn, 2007). The extent to which a message manages to attract attention is important, as attention is prerequisite to further effects (Lobinger, 2012).

Previous research clearly suggested that visuals outperform words when it comes to attracting people's attention (Bucher & Schumacher, 2006; Donsbach, 1991; Garcia & Stark, 1991; Holsanova, Rahm, & Holmqvist, 2006; Mendelson & Thorson, 2004; Pfau et al., 2006; Zillmann, Knobloch, & Yu, 2001). Photos showing faces and those that are emotionally involving seem particularly effective (Kanwisher, McDermott, & Chun, 1997; Knobloch, Hastall, Zillmann, & Callison, 2003; Levy, Hasson, & Malach, 2004; O'Toole, 2005; Parker, 2003; Zillmann et al., 2001). Scholars estimate that about 80% of newspaper readers notice visuals (Blum & Bucher, 1998), but only about 10%–20% acknowledge the text (Kroeber-Riel, 1996).

An array of eye-tracking studies substantiates this argument. In these studies, scholars use a special device to measure where people look and for how long, when exposed to a certain stimulus. The results obtained from this line of research are quite consistent. People's scanning of stimulus material is consistently interrupted when the eye encounters photos, especially, but also headlines (Barthelson, 2002; Bucher, 2008; Bucher & Schumacher, 2006; Holsanova et al., 2006; Küpper, 1990; McLellan & Steele, 2001; Stenfors, Morén, & Balkenius, 2003; Wolf & Grotta, 1985). Photos and headlines are among the most reliable "entry points" (Garcia & Stark, 1991, p. 1) for multimodal messages.

Visuals impact more than people's selection of few stimuli out of those demanding attention. They also have an effect on information processing in that visuals are processed before and faster than words (Gibson & Zillmann, 2000; Pfau et al., 2006). Scholars argue that visual information is processed about 6,000 times faster than words (Barry, 2005; Gazzaniga, 1992; Newell, 1990). At least four theories—the Dual Coding Theory (DCT) (Paivio, 1986), the Heuristic Systematic Model (HSM) (Chen & Chaiken, 1999), the Elaboration Likelihood Model (ELM) (Petty & Cacioppo, 1984), and the Limited Capacity Model (LCM) (Lang, 2000)—speak to this phenomenon.

First, Dual Coding Theory (Paivio, 1986) postulates that words and visuals are processed in interconnected subsystems dedicated to words or visuals, respectively. The verbal subsystem processes words one by one, logically and consciously (Gazzaniga, 1998; Rodriguez & Dimitrova, 2011), whereas the visual system processes visual cues immediately and unconsciously (Busselle & Bhandzic, 2011; Gordon, 2004; Müller, 2003; Paivio, 1979, 1986). Thus, the DCT proposes that the processing of verbal information is necessarily much slower than that of visual information.

Additionally, the Heuristic Systematic Model (Chen & Chaiken, 1999) and the Elaboration Likelihood Model (Petty & Cacioppo, 1984) shed some light on why visuals are processed before and faster than words. Though there are differences between these theories (see for a recent review Coleman & Wu, 2015), delving into them is beyond the purpose here. Suffice it to say that, notwithstanding the use of a different terminology, both theories posit that messages are processed either analytically or superficially. Superficial processing is inevitably quicker than analytical processing. To the extent that visuals are processed superficially, they will also be processed faster than words. It is important to note, however, that neither the HSM nor the ELM poses that visuals are processed superficially and words analytically. Instead, ability and motivation are key to whether or not a message will be further processed (see Lazard & Atkinson, 2015; Turner, Skubisz, Pandya, Silverman, & Austin, 2014). As Coleman and Wu (2015) put it, "If a picture attracts a person's attention and holds it, encouraging the viewer to think about what it contains, it will be processed centrally, with careful, rational thought" (p. 43).

Finally, the Limited Capacity Model (Lang, 2000) says that news in a video format—i.e., consisting of many modalities such as words, visuals, and sound—can overtax the processing system. The assumption is that visuals will impair the processing of words and other modalities (Noller, 1985; Posner, Nissen, & Klein, 1976). Visuals will be processed preferentially at the expense of words. The evidence for this is mixed. Some authors find that visually complex messages can overwhelm recipients to such a degree that they only attend to the visual components of the message while disregarding the verbal components (Southwell, 2005). Others find quite the opposite (Niederdeppe, Davis, Farrelly, & Yarsevich, 2007; Norris, Bailey, Bolls, & Wise, 2012). The authors of the two studies that seem to contradict the premise of the LCM acknowledge, however, that their stimuli may not have been as visually complex as those used in other LCM studies confirming Lang's (2000) hypothesis.

Memory and Recall

I have noted that multimodal messages are quite common. In this section, I turn to the way multimodality affects memory for the information conveyed. Previous studies suggest that multimodal messages can either increase or obstruct memory for and recall of the information conveyed. Which of these two scenarios kicks in depends mostly on whether the words and the visuals in a given message complement one another or conflict.

Previous studies found that adding congruent visuals to a verbal message increased the likelihood that audiences retained that information

(Pfau et al., 2006). "Audio-visual redundancy" research generally confirms this (Drew & Grimes, 1987; Grimes, 1991; Lang, 1995). Overall, visuals are better recalled and remembered than words. For example, in political communication, Bucy and Newhagen (1999) found that recall and memory for visual information on TV was at about 70%–80% but only at 55% for verbal information. In another study, participants were exposed to both audiovisual and audio-based TV news stories, and then asked to narrate what the story was about (Graber, 1990). It was found that visual themes were remembered twice as well as verbal themes; close-ups of people were especially memorable.

From this perspective, adding congruent visuals to a message can only improve memory and recall. Most scholars resort to the Dual Coding Theory to explain such findings (see above section), especially to the additivity hypothesis, which reads, "verbal and nonverbal codes corresponding to the same object (e.g., pictures and their names) can have additive effects on recall" (Paivio, 1991, p. 259).[1] The line of argument advanced by the proponents of Dual Coding is easy to follow: Visuals are better remembered than words, because they activate both the verbal and the visual subsystems and leave traces in both memory subsystems. This means visuals are coded twice, once in each subsystem. Words, on the other hand, mostly activate just the verbal subsystem and are coded only in this one subsystem. In short, visuals are double stored in memory, and this double-storing makes them more easily retrievable than words, which are only stored once, in just one memory subsystem (see also David, 2008). Adding congruent visuals to a verbal message is likely to render it more memorable.

Wide empirical support exists for this premise (Barlow & Wogalter, 1993; Chang, 2013; Frisch, Camerini, & Schulz, 2012; Perrault & Silk, 2014). A recent example is the study by Dixon, McKeever, Holton, Clarke, and Eosco (2015). This team of researchers found that misperceptions about an autism-vaccine link could be reduced when verbal information on the weight-of-evidence was accompanied by a photo of a group of scientists. The caption read "97% of physicians/medical scientists agree that vaccines do not cause autism" (Dixon et al., 2015, p. 645).

The extent to which audiences' memory and recall are aided by congruent messages appears to be moderated by personal characteristics. Specifically, individuals with low levels of literacy, prior knowledge, and formal education seem to benefit even more from verbal-visual congruence or redundancy than their counterparts (Entwistle & Williams, 2008; Houts, Doak, Doak, & Loscalzo, 2006; Mayer, 1997). Another personal characteristic of recipients moderating the benefit of having information presented verbally and visually is simply personal preference. Mendelson and Thorson (2004) proposed distinguishing between verbalizers and visualizers (see also Green & Schroeder, 1990). One assumption here was that visualizers benefit from verbal and visual information, whereas verbalizers not only do not learn from accompanying visuals but are disturbed by them (Mendelson & Thorson, 2004). Previous studies tend to support especially the first half of this assumption. For instance, two recent studies suggest that visualizers learn more from multimodal congruent messages, but that verbalizers are not disturbed by congruent visuals (Chang, 2013; Lazard & Atkinson, 2015).

Up to now, I have discussed the possible effects of congruent multimodal messages on recall and memory. The argument has been that visuals can increase recall and memory when words and visuals in a given message complement each other. But what are the effects of words and visuals conveying conflicting meanings?

Previous studies suggest that people tend to (mis-)remember information according to the visuals (Brosius, 1993; Graber, 2001; Grimes, 1991; Lang, 1995; Price & Feldman, 2008). This tendency is widely documented in the literature and is known as the Picture Superiority Effect (PSE) (Coleman & Wasike, 2004; Gibson & Zillmann, 2000; Graber, 1990; Grimes & Drechsel, 1996; Kobayashi, 1986; McBride & Dosher, 2002; Nelson & Castano, 1984; Paivio & Csapo, 1973; Wanta & Roark, 1994; Zillmann, Gibson, & Sargent, 1999).

One prolific line of research testing the premises of the PSE investigated the impact of smoking cues—smoking-related visuals—on viewers' encoding of anti-smoking arguments in PSAs. The findings suggest that smoking cues reduce smokers' interest in and memory for anti-smoking arguments in PSAs (e.g., Lee & Cappella, 2013).

To this point, the studies reviewed in this chapter contrasted either the effects of written/spoken words with that of still/moving images, or the effects of messages conveyed through one modality (words *or* visuals) with those conveyed through both multimodalities (words *and* visuals). Generally, framing scholars assumed that these studies' findings would hold true also when verbal frames are contrasted to visual frames[2] (e.g., Geise & Baden, 2015; Unz, 2007). Indeed, it appears plausible to assume that visual frames would yield more attention than verbal frames, would be processed faster and ahead of verbal frames, and would be remembered better than verbal frames. Consequently, when verbal frames and visual frames in one message contradict each other, recipients would be expected to attend to and remember the visual frame over the verbal one. When the same frame is conveyed verbally and visually in one message, recipients would pick up that respective frame more clearly and easily.

While only very few framing effects studies tested these assumptions specifically, their findings generally support the idea that previous research findings can be carried over to the realm of framing scholarship. For instance, Seo and Shen (2009) examined the effectiveness of message format (verbal vs. verbal-and-visual) and message frames (gain vs. loss) in PSAs on dental flossing and sunscreen use. The key finding of this study was that the verbal-and-visual loss frame generated more fear and persuasiveness than the verbal loss frame. Other scholars acknowledged this idea—that verbal frames would have to be congruent to visual frames in order to yield the desired effect—rather implicitly in their effects studies. This was, for example, the case in Cameron and Lee's (2006) study on how involvement moderated the effects of gain and loss framing. These authors used multimodal print PSAs as stimuli that consisted of "a headline, sub-headline, body copy and picture" (p. 11). They used a series of pretests/manipulation checks to ensure that their stimuli conveyed the same frame both verbally and visually. They justified their decision as follows: "If the contents are not equivalent between gain and loss stimuli, we may not know whether the differences of persuasion effects were elicited by message framing effects or discrepancies of the contents of the stimuli" (p. 11). In the end, their gain-framed message emphasized the benefits of quitting smoking (verbal) and showed "lungs filled with green trees" (visual); their loss-framed message addressed the health problems if one keeps smoking (verbal) and showed "lungs filled with dirty cigarette buds" (visual) (Cameron & Lee, 2006, p. 11).

Other studies tested the effects of frames in multimodal messages and designed their studies in such a way that the verbal frame was manipulated, but the visual was kept identical throughout conditions (e.g., O'Malley & Latimer-Cheung, 2013; Van Gorp, Vettehen, & Beentjes, 2009; Yan, 2015). These studies' findings are informative of the way various degrees of verbal-and-visual frame congruence impacted audiences, even though this was not formulated as a research goal in these studies. For instance, gain-framed messages were recalled best in a study using osteoporosis prevention print PSAs (O'Malley & Latimer-Cheung, 2013). While the authors did not describe the images used in the stimuli, they did state that the same image was used in the gain, loss, and neutral conditions. It is possible that the image conveyed a gain frame and that this was the reason why the strongest effects were obtained in this condition. In fact, this is perhaps one of the reasons why findings on the effects of gain vs. loss frames are mixed. For example, participants in a different study on junk food—again using the same visual across conditions—elaborated most on loss-framed PSAs (Yan, 2015). Again, it is conceivable that the image conveyed a loss frame and that the verbal-and-visual frame congruence explains the apparently contradicting results obtained by O'Malley and Latimer-Cheung (2013) and Yan (2015), respectively. A similar procedure was used in a study on the framing of asylum seekers as either victims or intruders (Van Gorp et al., 2009). These authors too paired an identical photograph with various verbal frames: victim, intruder, and mixed.[3] Upon exposure to the stimulus, study participants were asked to choose one of five possible interpretations of the photograph that best applied to them (e.g., "I feel pity for the persons on the photograph" or "I feel aversion and fear toward these persons"). Their analysis showed that the group exposed to the mixed frame interpreted the photograph in a more positive way than the group exposed to the intruder frame. As the photo showed four people in a camp, it is possible that it conveyed the intruder frame.

To my knowledge, the most detailed study to date on potential differences in framing effects by modality was conducted by Powell, Boomgaarden, De Swert, and de Vreese (2015). They found that when words and visuals were presented together, the verbal frame influenced opinions (i.e., military intervention) regardless of the accompanying image, whereas the visual frame influenced behavioral intention (i.e., discuss, donate, protest) irrespective of the accompanying verbal frame (Powell et al., 2015).

Notes

1 There is a possibility that, rather than aiding with memory and recall, this double-activation may overwhelm audiences, who might then only remember the information conveyed visually (see Limited Capacity Model above). However, in the case of congruent messages, where verbal and visual information convey the same message, the premise of this model does not weaken the argument that visuals improve memory and recall.

2 For instance, Unz (2007) expected that structural features such as camera angles would influence the cognitive processing of information and thus the framing of that issue. She relied, among others, on a study showing that camera angles influenced the attributions of causality (Lassiter, Geers, Munhall, Ploutz-Snyder, & Breitenbecher, 2002).

3 The assumption was that the verbal frame would suggest ways to interpret the polysemous photograph. This reminds of an older contention by Berger (1992) that "[t]he caption provides a handle, a means by which language, in the act of constructing a logical narrative, may reenter the space of the photograph" (p. 14).

3 Why so Few Integrative Framing Analyses?

The previous chapters were intended to clarify the importance of conducting verbal and visual framing analyses. This one is focused on three methodological challenges to this endeavor, as they may be responsible for the still very low number of integrative framing studies.

Approaches to Verbal Framing Analysis

Matthes and Kohring (2008) surveyed previous verbal framing studies for the techniques used to identify verbal frames (see also de Vreese & Lecheler, 2012). These authors classified studies based on their use of one of the following approaches: (1) hermeneutic, (2) linguistic, (3) manual holistic, (4) computer-assisted, and (5) deductive. Additionally they proposed a sixth approach which they named (6) manual clustering (see Matthes & Kohring, 2008; Figure 3.1).

The studies classified by Matthes and Kohring (2008) as taking a (1) hermeneutic approach are those that connect frames in news stories with broader cultural elements. I would argue that Van Gorp (2007) has written some of the most important hermeneutic studies to date. This author credits Gamson and colleagues for inspiration (Gamson, 1989; Gamson & Lasch, 1983; Gamson & Modigliani, 1989).

Van Gorp (2007) assumes that frames in culture get embedded in a text during the framing process. Scholars using this author's approach must identify the so-called identity kits of frames. Each identity kit contains framing and reasoning devices (see Figure 3.2). Framing devices, such as metaphors and catchphrases, are manifest. Reasoning devices, on the other hand, can be either manifest or latent and are known as roots, consequences, and appeals to principle.[1] These devices act as cues for the cultural phenomena, inviting a reading of the text through this lens (Johnson-Cartee, 2004).

This distinction between manifest and latent devices is important, as a latent reasoning device—i.e., one that is not explicitly stated in a text but which is known to the audience—can be activated during the interpretation process of the reader (Van Gorp, 2005, 2007). Entman (1993) even argued that the whole frame can be activated by a single prominent device, provided the frame is well-known to audiences. Thus, researchers are advised by Van Gorp (2010) to ascertain the "weight" of the frame in each news piece. This

DOI: 10.4324/9781315171456-3

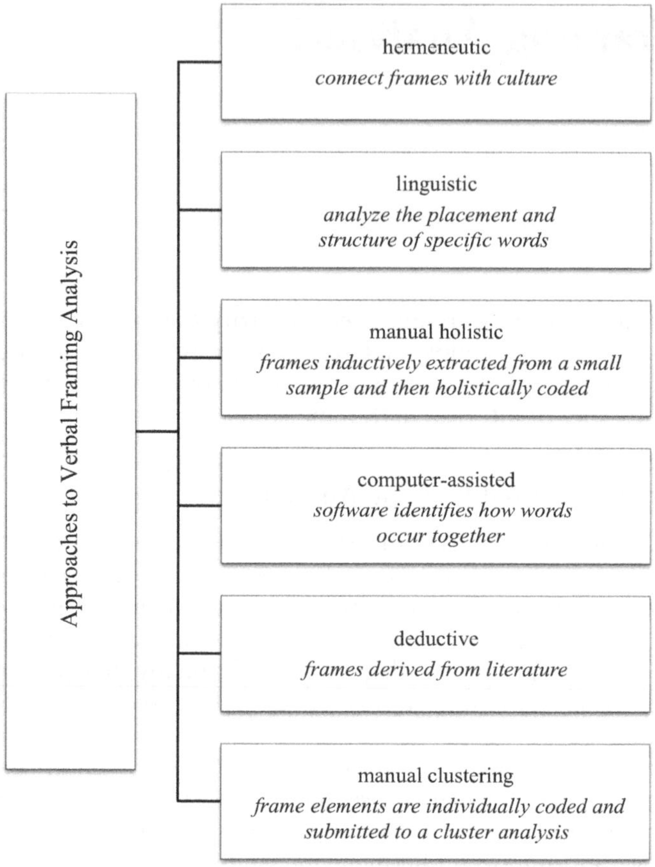

Figure 3.1 Approaches to Verbal Framing Analysis.

is done by counting how many framing and reasoning devices appeared in each text. The assumption is that the higher their number, the higher the chance that they will evoke a schema in the mind of the reader that is in line with the frame to which the devices refer. Matthes (2007) had implemented this advice by distinguishing between explicit and implicit frames based on the number of devices identified in a text. Specifically, Matthes (2007) assumed that two devices cuing the same frame in a text suffice for asserting that frame's existence in that text.

The main strengths of the (1) hermeneutic approach, and especially of Van Gorp's approach, are that it allows a distinction between content and frames, it aligns well with prevalent frame definitions by emphasizing culture, and it is constructionist (see Van Gorp, 2005, 2007). I would add that, because of its explicit consideration of the underlying culture, this approach may well reveal frames generalizable to topics other than those analyzed. Yet Van Gorp concedes that his approach is very time consuming

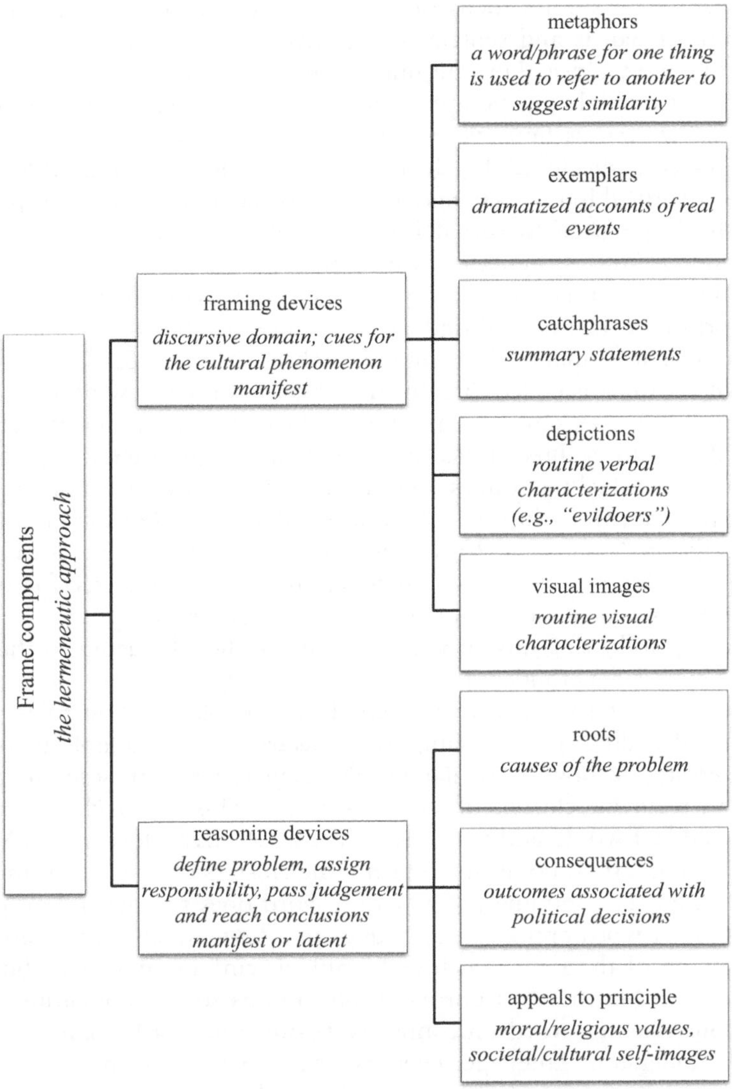

Figure 3.2 Frame Components according to the Hermeneutic Approach.

and potentially subjective. Matthes and Kohring's (2008) reservations regarding this approach also include subjectivity and cost, to which they add lack of transparency over explaining precisely how the frames were identified. However, I would argue that the last criticism does not apply to Van Gorp's work. This approach can also be criticized for conceptualizing visuals only as framing devices; the possibility that visuals convey frames by themselves—and that the visual is a modality in its own right also when it comes to framing—was not acknowledged.

I now turn to the discussion of framing studies taking a (2) linguistic approach. Such studies focus on word choice and on the placement and structure of words and sentences in a given text. As such, this approach cannot be used in visual or multimodal analyses, at least not without major adjustments. The linguistic approach allows an in-depth analysis of some texts, but a serious limitation is that it is not suitable for large samples (Matthes & Kohring, 2008). In my view, an additional limitation is that frames identified in this way may be hard to generalize to other topics.

A third approach to verbal framing analysis included in Matthes and Kohring's (2008) systematization is the (3) manual holistic approach. Scholars striking this path identify frames by means of a qualitative analysis of a portion of the material (inductively) and then code the frames as holistic variables in a quantitative content analysis (Matthes & Kohring, 2008). The whole frame is coded directly and at once. In the view of Matthes and Kohring (2008), this approach is not problematic per se, but its reliability and validity are a direct function of scholars' transparency regarding the way they identified the frames. Indeed, when transparency is not a problem, this approach can be just as valid and reliable as nonholistic ones (David, Atun, Fille, & Monterola, 2011). I would argue that a further advantage of this approach arises out of its closeness to the material selected for analysis. Also, this approach allows an effective use of resources.

Scholars following any of the three approaches discussed to this point used human coders to identify frames. Those using the (4) computer-assisted approach resort to software instead. Here, scholars define rules for the automated coding of large samples of electronically available texts. They are interested in how particular words occur together in some texts; they interpret recurring clusters of words as frames. This approach is considered very reliable. I would add that it is also cost-effective. However, as Matthes and Kohring (2008) point out, interpreting clusters of words as frames may not be valid. The framing potency of a word does not depend only on its repetition. A word appearing only once in a text can contribute greatly to the framing of the issue—such as "Frankenstein" in an article about biogenetics (see Matthes & Kohring, 2008). But as software identifies frames based on recurring words, it cannot (yet) substitute for human coders able to fully understand language. There is also a chance that the frames identified in this way will not be generalizable to other topics.

The last approach identified by Matthes and Kohring (2008) in previous publications is the (5) deductive approach. These studies theoretically derive frames from the literature and code them in standard content analysis (Matthes & Kohring, 2008). This is the only approach in the typology that is not inductive. It is also the only one that allows the identification of frames that are likely to be identified on other topics, too. Yet Matthes and Kohring (2008) acknowledge the difficulty of knowing exactly which frames one will encounter in a sample. There is a risk that researchers will overlook unanticipated frames. Despite these limitations, I would argue that deductive framing studies contribute to theory building in a unique way, given that they allow scholars to build on others' work. For instance, in health communication, Clarke et al.'s medical, lifestyle, and political/economy frames have allowed scholars to compare the news framing of various health conditions using the same benchmarks (e.g., Clarke & Binns, 2006; Ye & Ward, 2010).

In their quest for a reliable and valid alternative to the five approaches reviewed above, Matthes and Kohring (2008) proposed the (6) manual-clustering approach. Here, frames were conceptualized as latent constructs revealed through the clustering of specific frame elements separately coded. The frame elements—problem definition, causal interpretation, moral evaluation, and treatment recommendation—were drawn from Entman's (1993) definition.

Matthes and Kohring (2008) argue that their approach is more reliable than holistic ones, because frame elements are more manifest than entire frames and thus easier to code reliably. Yet, as already mentioned above, David and colleagues (2011) demonstrated that this isn't necessarily the case. Perhaps the most important merit of this approach is that it reduces the chances that coders will be influenced by their own schemas. This is because they code single frame elements without knowing how the elements relate to one another, rather than coding entire frames, where they would run the risk of forcing the material into a familiar frame. For these reasons, it seems to me that the manual-clustering approach made a solid methodological contribution to building framing theory.

This approach is not without its drawbacks, however. In my opinion, the most serious shortcomings are related to the use of a cluster analysis, given that the entire article was often used as the unit of analysis. This implies that researchers must use a limited number of variables for frame elements and a limited number of frames altogether. But as Matthes and Kohring (2008) also acknowledge, texts are likely to contain more than one frame. Thus, much of the information available risks getting lost in the cluster analysis. Finally, I would add that when frames are identified as closely to the research material as proposed by this approach, they do not stand a very good chance of being identified in studies on other topics. Every research project choosing this approach will likely propose new frames, which runs counter to the key idea that frames occur over and over again, independent of topics.

Approaches to Visual Framing Analysis

According to Fahmy, Bock, and Wanta (2014), framing is "an obvious theoretical framework for visual communication" (p. 2). Indeed, many studies analyzing visuals cite framing in their theory sections. While the number of visual framing studies pales by comparison to that of verbal framing studies,[2] many scholars have devoted attention to visual framing in the last decade.

Rodriguez and Dimitrova's (2011) effort to survey previous visual framing studies for the techniques used to identify visual frames was much needed. I think this publication does for visual framing research what Matthes and Kohring's (2008) did for verbal framing scholarship—that is, it reviews existing literature and classifies studies based on the way scholars operationalize frames. Both Rodriguez and Dimitrova (2011) and Matthes and Kohring (2008) can assist scholars in finding the right approach for answering their research questions.

In this section, I briefly review each of the four approaches identified by Rodriguez and Dimitrova (2011): (1) denotative, (2) connotative, (3) symbolic-semiotic, and (4) ideological (see Figure 3.3). Also, I add methodological insight to each of the four categories, drawing on landmark publications on visual framing (especially Coleman, 2010; Geise, Lobinger, & Brantner, 2013; Grabe & Bucy, 2009) and recent empirical studies.

(1) Denotative studies categorize content in broad categories understood as frames. According to Rodriguez and Dimitrova (2011), scholars using this approach sometimes resort to the words surrounding a visual to derive meaning, but purely visual framing studies are more typical. By contrast, (2) connotative studies extract meaning from symbols and visual metaphors, such as crosses, flags, or ribbons (see Rodriguez & Dimitrova, 2011).

Denotative studies can be classified further into deductive and inductive studies (see Geise et al., 2013; Figure 3.3). Deductive denotative studies are those in which researchers identify frames in previous literature and investigate the extent to which these frames appear in their sample. Inductive denotative studies derive frames from scholars' own observations of the

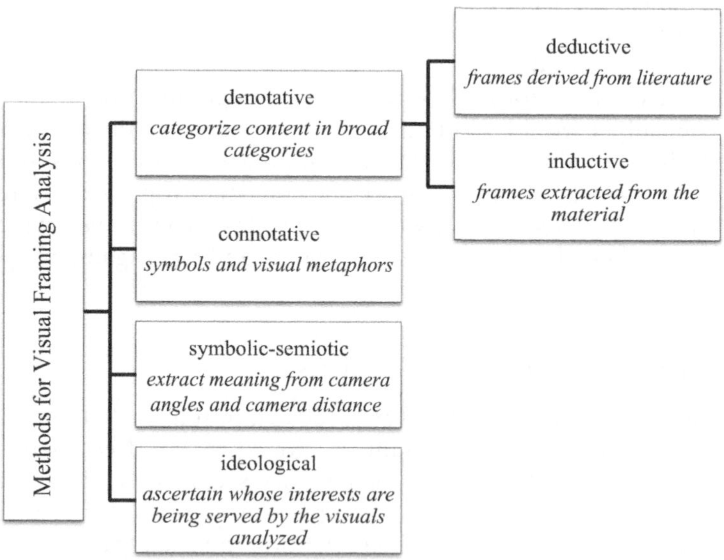

Figure 3.3 Approaches to Visual Framing Analysis.

material sampled for analysis. Such studies are common when the previous literature offers little guidance on what to expect in the material.

To better illustrate the distinction between inductive and deductive studies, I briefly present two studies on the visual reporting of the 2003 toppling of the Saddam Hussein statue during the U.S.-led invasion of Iraq. The first visual framing study of these events was conducted by Aday, Cluverius, and Livingston (2005). These authors did not find any guidance in previous studies regarding the frames conveyed by visuals like those in their sample. Thus, they proceeded inductively, merging visuals into categories based on the similarity of their content. Among others, they proposed that photos showing triumphant people convey a victory frame. Two years later, in her analysis of the visual framing of the same event in a different sample, Fahmy (2007) relied on Aday et al.'s (2005) work to operationalize the frames she expected to find, including the previously identified victory frame. In this way, Fahmy's (2007) study was deductive. Many more deductive denotative studies exist (e.g., Borah, 2009; Schwalbe, Silcock, & Keith, 2008). They look for established frames such as conflict and human interest. Inductive studies occur but are less common (Griffin, 2004; Smith, 2006).

The content of visuals is surely important for visual framing analyses. Such analyses "can reveal much about the organizing ideas and the visual framing choices of … newspapers, [as] the visual coverage … represents selections from possible photographs that have been published at different stages of the news making process" (Fahmy & Kim, 2008, p. 449). Yet despite this unquestionable merit of content-based framing analyses of the visual, documenting visual content may not provide sufficient basis for turning a visual study into a visual framing study (see Coleman, 2010). After all, describing words' content is not enough for verbal framing analyses either (Reese, 2007). More insights can be gathered from symbolic-semiotic perspectives, to which I turn next.

Scholars investigating visual framing from a (3) symbolic-semiotic perspective are interested in the somewhat abstract aspects of visuals, such as camera angles, in studies of both moving (Grabe, 1996) and still images (Moriarty & Popovich, 1991). Scholars extract latent meaning mainly regarding power and social distance from information gathered in this fashion (Coleman, 2010). Alternatively, researchers can analyze the (4) ideological level of images to tackle questions of power in a more holistic, less specific way.

I now address the three aspects of visual communication that previous literature identifies as the most relevant to framing from a symbolic-semiotic perspective—namely, camera angle, camera distance, and nonverbal behavior (see Table 3.1).

Camera angles and camera distances are known in the literature as structural features (Coleman, 2010) or as visual information packaging (Grabe & Bucy, 2009). Few studies in our discipline at large analyze camera angles and camera distances (see Coleman, 2010). Nonetheless, there appears to be much potential for such analyses, as I discuss below. The preferred contexts are war/catastrophe media coverage (Borah, 2009; Fahmy, 2004b; King & Lester, 2005; Parry, 2011) and political campaigns (Banning & Coleman, 2009; Biocca, 2014; Grabe, 1996).

The *camera angle* refers to the placement of the camera higher or lower than the person being photographed (Bell & Milic, 2002). Here, photographers, photojournalists, and camera people can opt for a high-, low-, or eye-level angle. In a high-angle shot, the camera looks down on the subject. In a low-angle shot, the camera is located below the subject. Finally, for an eye-level shot, the camera is placed at the eye level of the person being photographed. Variations in camera angles can affect the way the subject is perceived. Researchers typically interpret these angles as summarized in Table 3.1, with eye-level and low shots conveying more power than high shots (Banning & Coleman, 2009; Bell & Milic, 2002; Berger, 1981; Coleman, 2010; Grabe & Bucy, 2009; Jewitt & Oyama, 2012; Messaris, 1997). It is important to note that these are not necessarily the meanings of these angles; it is impossible for anyone to say what they mean exactly (Jewitt & Oyama, 2012, p. 152). But when photographers opt for a certain angle, they considerably reduce the field of possible meanings viewers are likely to extract from the photos. For instance, perceiving a person as powerful is much more likely when viewing a photo using a low angle than one using a high angle (see Table 3.1).

Camera distance refers to the distance from the camera of the person being photographed or recorded (Berger, 1981; Messaris, 1997; Shook, 2000). Here, the main options professionals can choose from are (extreme) close-up, medium shot, and long shot. Close-ups and extreme close-ups are images showing little more than the face of the subject. Medium shots begin to reveal more of the environment and show the face and torso of the person depicted. Long shots show up to the full body of the subject and some of the surrounding environment. In other words, variations in camera distance make the subject seem closer to or farther from the viewer both spatially and socially (see Coleman, 2010; Grabe & Bucy, 2009). Variations in camera distance can affect the perceived social distance between viewer and subject by varying the degree of spatial distance. The ways scholars understand these angles are summarized in Table 3.1 (based on a review by Grabe & Bucy, 2009), with close-ups conveying intimacy, medium shots being neutral, and long shots indicating social distance. Here, too, it is important to understand that a certain camera distance setting may—but does not necessarily—convey social proximity or distance.

Professional training informs prospective photographers, photojournalists, and camera persons about the technical choices at their disposal and how they can be used to convey a certain meaning (Grabe, Lang, & Zhao, 2003; Schwartz, 1992). These professionals seem well aware of the effects their choice of camera angle and camera distance can have on audiences (Graber, 1987; Kepplinger, 1982). As variations in camera angle and shot distance reproduce human interaction (Messaris, 1994), "manipulations in these characteristics can produce changes in viewers' evaluations, and the perceptions they create are not neutral" (Coleman, 2010, p. 248). Thus, according to Coleman (2010), structural features represent "an important aspect of visual framing" (p. 248). Additionally, when variations in structural features occur intentionally, they may indicate bias (see Grabe & Bucy, 2009). This would be the case, for instance, when a TV station openly endorsing a political candidate constantly depicts her using low camera angles and/or close-ups—while opting for high camera angles and/or long camera distances for her adversaries.

As mentioned above, symbolic-semiotic studies are not only interested in camera angle and distance, but also in nonverbal behavior and the interactions among the people depicted.

Most studies analyzing *nonverbal behavior* are conducted in political communication; the focus is on political candidates. Researchers pay attention to posture, hands, and facial expressions, among other things (see Table 3.1 for a full list and likely connotations among viewers; see also Coulson, 2004; Kress & van Leeuwen, 1996; Mignault & Chaudhuri, 2003). Coleman and Wu (2015) identified facial expressions as the most important type of nonverbal information (p. 102). Studies investigating nonverbal behavior use either broad or specific categories. For instance, Coleman and Wu (2015) assessed the overall appearance of political candidates with an inclusive variable containing demeanor, delivery, attitude, and facial expressions. Grabe and Bucy (2009) coded facial expressions with the help of various micro variables registering variations in mouth corners, teeth visibility, frowns, and so on. As both studies reported high reliability coefficients, both approaches seem valid.

The nonverbal behavior of the people depicted can be very informative for scholars interested in the framing of these people. Members of the audience form impressions of others based on their nonverbal behavior, especially based on their facial expressions (see for a recent review Dan & Coleman, 2014). Photographers, photojournalists, and camera people choose images conveying specific behaviors. It is likely that the nonverbal behavior shown in the images chosen for air or print highlights some parts of people's personalities while obscuring others. In this way, the nonverbal behavior of the people shown contributes to their framing.

Finally, scholars can also analyze the interaction between the person of interest and the other people visible in the images. (This only applies to images showing more than one person.) Analyzing the interaction among the subjects in an image informs about the power dynamics among them. This is important to the framing of people, as it shows whose interests are being served and who has symbolic power over whom in the context analyzed (see Table 3.1).

Two aspects are important here, positioning and action. Kress and van Leeuwen (1996) explained how photos showing more than one person convey hierarchy through the positioning of the people relative to one another.

Table 3.1 The Symbolic-Semiotic Approach to Visual Framing

Type	*Category*	*Variation*	*Connotation*
Structural features	Camera angle = the placement of the camera compared to the subject	High angle shot = camera looks down on the subject	The viewer looks down on the subject; conveys weakness of the subject by comparison to the viewer. The viewer gets the impression that s/he is more powerful than the subject.
		Low angle shot = camera is located below the subject	The viewer looks up on the subject; conveys power and dominance of the subject over the viewer. The viewer gets the impression that the subject is more powerful than himself/herself.
		Eye-level shot = camera is located at the eye-level of the subject	Conveys parity between viewer and subject.
	Camera distance = the distance of the subject from the camera	Extreme close-up = just the face of the subject is visible; chin or forehead may be visually cut off	A high level of intimacy between viewer and subject is generated; the privacy of the subject is invaded. This may discomfit the viewer and lead to negative attitudes toward the subject.
		Close-up = face and shoulders of the subject are visible; chin or forehead may be visually cut off; breast area not visible	Intimacy between subject and viewer is created. This may lead to positive attitudes toward the subject.
		Medium shot = face and breast area of the subject are visible	A comfortable distance between viewer and subject is established; neutral.
		Long shot = more than the face and the breast area of the subject are visible (i.e., waist, buttocks, hips, legs, and/or feet are visible)	A high level of distance is created. The viewer may feel disconnected from the subject and pay attention to the details surrounding the subject. May lead to negative or less positive attitudes toward the subject.
Nonverbal behavior	Activity	Active = speaking, shaking hands, waving, etc.	Positive
		Passive = listening, reading, etc.	Negative
	Posture	Standing tall and upright	Positive
		Bowed, slumped, or leaning	Negative

Type	*Category*	*Variation*	*Connotation*
	Arms	Held at shoulder height or above	Positive
		At rest, the sides, or folded	Negative
	Hands	Gesturing or doing something	Positive
		At rest	Negative
	Eyes	Looking directly at the camera or someone	Positive
		Looking indirectly, up or down, or being closed	Negative
	Overall appearance = demeanor, delivery, attitude, and facial expression	Smiling, confident, relaxed, enthusiastic, cheerful	Positive
		Angry, tense, tired, tentative, unhappy, worried, lethargic, or passive	Negative
		Intent, passive, or has a serious expression	Neutral
	Position = the positioning of the subjects to one another	Symmetrical = subjects are located at the same level	Equality among subjects
		Asymmetrical = one/more subjects are located above others	The subject located higher is placed at the top of the hierarchy, whereas the subject located lower is at its bottom.
	Action = acting or acted upon?	Target of others' actions	Passive, weak, dependent
		Doers	Vibrant, strong

Note: Subject = the person depicted.

Symmetrical positioning suggests equality. Asymmetrical positioning places the one located higher at the top of the hierarchy and the one located lower at its bottom. For example, a photo showing a person sitting while other people stand places the person sitting at a lower rank than those standing. Similarly, a photo showing a person addressing a crowd from a stage symbolically places that person at a higher rank than the audience.

Action refers to whether the subject is acting or being acted upon (Bell & Milic, 2002; Kress & van Leeuwen, 1996). The question is: Who does something to or for whom? This serves as an indicator of self-determination and social power. Specifically, passive, weak, dependent people are targets of others' action, while vibrant and strong individuals act themselves. There is some overlap between this measure and some measures of nonverbal behavior in terms of how the information gathered is to be interpreted.

Table 3.1 summarizes the literature reviewed and discussed above. I argue that most visual framing studies to date can be categorized in one of the four groups proposed by Rodriguez and Dimitrova (2011). Yet as Coleman (2010) rightly pointed out, visual framing scholars can combine several approaches. For example, Grabe and Bucy (2009) combined three of the four approaches to visual framing in their study of political candidates. The presence or absence of each character frame of interest was signaled to the authors by visual characteristics pertaining to content (denotative approach) and symbols (connotative approach). These authors had also analyzed nonverbal behavior and structural features (symbolic-semiotic approach), though they had not explicitly attributed them a framing function.

Approaches to Integrative Framing Analysis

Across disciplines, researchers have come to agree that when a message consists of words and visuals, both modalities should be included in the empirical analysis (e.g., Rose, 2012). While framing scholars generally expressed agreement with this view (e.g., Coleman, 2010; Geise et al., 2013), very few of their studies actually analyzed both modalities.

Despite the low number of studies, the identification of similarities and differences in the way empirical research was conducted is possible. To date, most of these studies focused on the media coverage; topics included environmental matters (Dotson, Jacobson, Kaid, & Carlton, 2012; Liebler & Bendix, 1996; Wessler, Wozniak, Hofer, & Lück, 2016), unemployment (Dan & Ihlen, 2011b), terrorist attacks (Reynolds & Barnett, 2003), elections (Dan & Iorgoveanu, 2013; Khamis & Mahmoud, 2013; Van Hoof, Takens, & Oegema, 2010), the asylum issue (Van Gorp, 2005), military operations (Entman, 1991), Sub-Saharan Africa (Mellese & Müller, 2012), and sporting events (Huang & Fahmy, 2011).

At first sight, the procedures chosen in this body of work seem rather homogenous: Across studies, (1) merely one research instrument was used for both modalities. Consequently, (2) analysts collected data from both modalities at once. Notwithstanding these similarities, the procedures differed in one key aspect, namely (3) the way scholars approached the interplay between the verbal and visual modalities. The next sections present an in-depth discussion of these similarities and differences, together with a critical appraisal.

Obviously, when data are to be collected from multimodal material, research instruments must entail variables taking into account the specific characteristics of each modality. Thus, the fact that studies to date have developed (1) codebooks containing variables referring to both the verbal and the visual components of the material is not surprising. What is surprising, however, is that *just one* research instrument *for both* modalities was used in these studies. The main benefit of this strategy is that it can be time-saving. However, as outlined below, its drawbacks outweigh its benefits by far.

This 2-in-1 strategy is likely the reason why only a limited number of visual characteristics were accounted for in the verbal-and-visual framing studies published so far. Specifically, analysts only acknowledged image content; aspects such as nonverbal behavior or structural features were not taken into account. This sole focus on content resembles the way words are typically analyzed, and it was perhaps an attempt to make visuals more tangible by employing methods known from the more familiar realm of words. While this is understandable, simply adapting methods for the analysis of words to that of visuals is not a viable solution. This is because much of the meaning conveyed by visuals is lost (see also Graber, 1990; Lobinger, 2012). In addition, this disregards high-performance methods specifically developed for this purpose over decades of visual communication scholarship (e.g., Barnhurst, Vari, & Rodriguez, 2004; Messaris, 2003; Rose, 2012; Van Leeuwen & Jewitt, 2001). Unfortunately, many framing studies acknowledging visuals are conducted without connecting to visual communication theories in a significant way (see also McWhirter & Hoffman-Goetz, 2014).

Furthermore, by conducting an elaborate verbal analysis, but only a hasty visual one, most of these scholars conceded a hierarchy of modalities as true that is no longer thought to be accurate (with words at the top and visuals at the bottom). This means that the verbal content was studied as the "real" venue of frames and that visuals only interested as add-ons, as ornament to the verbal frames. Accordingly, most studies to date devised *framing* variables for the words, but limited themselves to *content-related* variables for the visuals.[3] Analyses designed in this way can only reveal how *verbal* frames co-occurred with image content (Dan & Ihlen, 2011b; Dotson et al., 2012; Van Hoof et al., 2010; Wessler et al., 2016).

Some examples are in order here. In one study self-described as analyzing verbal and visual frames (Mellese & Müller, 2012), the authors did not actually code visual information but made inferences on the visuals by analyzing the photo captions. They stated that "[o]nly captions were considered when coding visuals, neither the associated text nor the visual motif of the respective press photograph" was coded/analyzed (pp. 213–214). This means that the authors had not accounted for meanings conveyed by the visuals themselves, and that valuable information was lost because the few words in a caption aren't likely to convey the multiple meanings in a photograph. The codebook we used in Dan and Ihlen (2011b) contained a wide array of verbal framing variables relevant to the unemployment issue. From the visuals, however, we only extracted information regarding socio-demographic characteristics of the subjects, the setting, and the (vice) behavior shown. Accordingly, we could only identify which subjects, settings, and behaviors were depicted when a certain verbal frame was conveyed. One such finding was that a rather sympathetic verbal framing of the unemployed was paired with images of idle men with an alcohol problem (Dan & Ihlen, 2011b). Huang and Fahmy's (2011) study was a notable exception from the trend of reproducing the outdated hierarchy of modalities in empirical research, as these authors investigated the interplay between *visual* frames and text.

The characteristics of the research instrument are consequential for (2) data collection. Accordingly, judging from the methodological information offered in these studies, analysts were exposed to the multimodal material and asked to collect data from both modalities at once. In her seminal chapter, Coleman (2010) advised scholars interested in verbal and visual framing to conduct two separate framing analyses in one study: one for words, one for visuals. (Obviously, the two data sets resulting from this procedure would have to be re-connected during data analysis.) Despite this publication's great influence on framing research, no study to date has attempted to implement this advice. A possible explanation was suggested by Coleman (2010) herself, who characterized such endeavors as a "daunting task" (p. 235). While this is likely to be an accurate representation, the fact that studies to date used just one research instrument for both modalities is very unfortunate because this runs the risk that the data misrepresent the material.

Considering the literature reviewed in Chapter 2, asking coders to extract information from words alone even though they see the accompanying visuals (and vice versa) is a source of error. Coders' attention is very likely to be directed to the visuals, which they would process faster and ahead of words. Furthermore, when conflicting interpretations of the issue at hand are conveyed in the two modalities, coders would remember the visuals over the words (see Chapter 2). Recognizing this source of error is not an expression of a lack of confidence in coders. Rather, it is an acknowledgement of the fact that they, like anybody else, are subject to processing biases that favor visuals over words. Thus, these studies would have been much more accurate had the authors conducted two separate framing analyses of just the words and just the visuals and combined the results of the two analyses in a third step.

I now move to the discussion of differences in the way integrative framing analyses were conducted. As already mentioned, studies differed with respect to (3) the way scholars approached the interplay between the verbal and visual modalities. While this is something some researchers did not address or only did so in passing (e.g., Entman, 1991; Liebler & Bendix, 1996; Reynolds & Barnett, 2003), details are offered in some studies (Dan & Ihlen, 2011b; Dotson et al., 2012; Huang & Fahmy, 2011; Van Hoof et al., 2010; Wessler et al., 2016). This information reveals that the paths chosen to determine the interplay between the modalities were quite diverse.

Van Hoof et al. (2010) calculated the percentage of sentences in a news story where one element of the verbal frame (e.g., an actor involved in the issue) was shown. In our study on elections coverage, we used an index to identify frames consisting of both words and visuals (Dan & Iorgoveanu, 2013). Wessler et al. (2016) adopted a similar approach as we did, but they went one step further: These authors put both verbal and visual elements into a joint cluster analysis—in an adaptation of the manual clustering approach discussed above (Matthes & Kohring, 2008). Their goal was to "uncover salient patterns of textual-visual compositions" by showing how elements of verbal frames were arranged to visual content (p. 426). In other words, their cluster analysis "reconstruct[ed] which pictorial elements [were] typically combined with which text-based issue frames" (p. 429).

Such explicit discussions of the interplay between words and visuals go into the right direction. Moving forward, a more elaborate way to compare verbal frames to visual frames is needed. In the words of Wessler and colleagues (2016), scholars must engage into a "thorough investigation of … logico-semantic relations between image and text," seen as able to "further illuminate how exactly a multimodal frame is built in the news" (p. 441). They propose using Martinec and Salway's (2005) typology as a starting point.

As for the findings obtained with regard to the interplay: They were mixed. Some studies found low congruence between the modalities (Van Hoof et al., 2010; Liebler & Bendix, 1996; Mellese & Müller, 2012; Dan & Ihlen, 2011b), and others found high congruence (Entman, 1991; Reynolds & Barnett, 2003).

Several explanations are conceivable for these differences. First, the topics investigated by Entman (1991) and Reynolds and Barnett (2003) were—unlike those investigated in the other studies—matters of life or death. It is possible that journalists pay more attention to congruence because of this. Journalistic culture may also have played a role. Quite telling in this regard is the study by Huang and Fahmy (2011). These authors examined visual frames and their rapport to the captions in the media coverage of the 2008 Olympic torch relay in US and Chinese newspapers. In Chinese newspapers, where the torch relay was visually presented as a success, captions matched the visual frame. However, this was not the case in US newspapers, which were more likely to use captions highlighting protests against the torch relay, something that was different from the visual content of the images.

The studies reviewed in this chapter laid the foundation work for integrative framing studies. Still, there is much more work to be done, and methodological guidance in this regard is still sorely needed. My thoughts on how to conduct such analyses can be found in Chapter 5; they are put to a test in Chapter 6.

Interim Summary and Some General Remarks

This chapter presented six approaches to verbal framing analyses, five to visual framing analyses, and two to integrative framing analyses. A summary of the strengths and weakness of each approach can be found in Table 3.2.

Some general remarks regarding the juxtaposition of approaches in Table 3.2 are in order.

First, there is a wide array of approaches. This is certainly a blessing, as there is no such thing as too much methodological advice. Still, scholars must determine anew which approach is most suitable for each study. Each of them emphasizes different aspects of communication; the scholar must determine which are most relevant to the framing of the people or issues at hand (see also Entman, 1991, p. 8). For instance, the aspects accounted for by means of the symbolic-semiotic approach are very likely more relevant to the framing of people than to the framing of issues.

But how should scholars choose the appropriate approaches for their studies?

The review above suggested that some approaches have more weaknesses than others, but they appear to resonate with researchers nonetheless. Thus, scholars do not seem to choose an approach on the basis of graphic rating scales alone.

I argue this decision may be influenced by additional factors, including (1) scholars' notion of frames, (2) scholars' methodological preferences, (3) cost-benefit calculations, and (4) efforts toward methodological triangulation.

I expect that (1) scholars' notion of frames affects their choice of an analytical approach as follows: Those understanding frames as recurring patterns of interpretation—thus those interested in generic frames—are more likely to opt for a deductive approach. In verbal framing analyses, the approaches most suitable to this view are surely the deductive and the hermeneutic approaches. The manual-clustering approach could also be adjusted to meet these scholars' requirements. Their counterpart in visual framing analyses would be the denotative deductive approach. In turn, those who think of frames as issue-specific constructs would prefer inductive approaches instead (i.e., any of those summarized in Table 3.2 except the denotative [visual], the deductive [verbal], and the hermeneutic [verbal] approaches).

I also believe that (2) scholars' inclination toward qualitative, quantitative, or critical methods is likely to affect their choice of approaches to use in framing analyses.[4] Researchers' preference for qualitative, quantitative, or critical work is often very clear, even though the number of those clearly

Table 3.2 Strengths and Weaknesses of Previous Approaches

Level of Analysis	*Approach*	*Strengths*	*Weaknesses*
Verbal	*Hermeneutic* = frames as linked to culture; identified with the aid of identity kits (framing devices like metaphors and reasoning devices like appeals to principle)	• Complies with key frame definitions; constructionist • Generalizable frames • In-depth analyses	• Subjective • Time consuming • Possibly lack of transparency • Visuals only as part of verbal frames
	Linguistic = frames as word choice and placement	• In-depth analyses	• Time consuming • Nongeneralizable frames • No visual frames, though content could be categorized automatically
	Manual holistic = frames are identified qualitatively in a subsample and coded holistically in the rest of the sample	• Close to the material • Cost-effective	• Possibly low reliability • Possibly low validity • Nongeneralizable frames
	Computer-assisted = software identifies clusters of words interpreted as frames	• High reliability • Cost-effective	• Low validity • Nongeneralizable frames
	Deductive = frames are derived from previous studies and coded in standard content analysis	• Generalizable frames • Contributes to theory building	• Unexpected frames may be overlooked • Difficult to establish frames for analysis
	Manual clustering = frames are split into frame elements which are coded separately in standard content analysis	• High reliability • High validity	• Low number of variables needed for cluster-analysis • Nongeneralizable frames • Unit of analysis: just one frame per text
Visual	*Denotative inductive* = visuals are grouped in broad categories based on their content; categories are derived from one's own sample	• High reliability • Close to the material • Cost-effective	• In itself not sufficient • Nongeneralizable frames
	Denotative deductive = visuals are grouped in broad categories based on their content, as suggested by previous literature	• High reliability • Generalizable frames • Contributes to theory building • Cost-effective	• In itself not sufficient • Unexpected frames may be overlooked

(*Continued*)

Level of Analysis	*Approach*	*Strengths*	*Weaknesses*
	Connotative = extract meaning from symbols and visual metaphors	• Typically visual measure • Informs about latent meaning	• Symbols and visual metaphors may not be relevant to the framing of all issues and people
	Symbolic-semiotic = latent meaning is extracted from camera angles, camera distance and nonverbal behavior (see Table 3.1)	• Typically visual measure • Informs about latent meaning • Particularly relevant to the framing of people	• Some authors categorize some characteristics as elements of bias, not of framing • Possibly not suitable for the analysis of issues
	Ideological = a generalized way to assess whose interests are served through visuals	• Tackles questions of power	• Possibly lack of transparency • Threats to reliability • Overlap with the symbolic-semiotic approach
Integrative (verbal and visual)	*Simultaneously* = verbal and visual frames are identified at the same time	• Time-saving • Less intimidating	• Unacceptable amalgamation of words and visuals in research instruments and during data collection • Disregards that visuals are processed and stored separately
	Separately = verbal and visual frames are identified one after another and reconnected in the analysis	• Acknowledges previous research on the way visuals are processed and stored • Acknowledges visuals as a modality different than words • Higher reliability and a better representation of the material as coders are not influenced by words when coding visuals and vice versa	• More time consuming • There is no formula that can be used to explicitly compute the ratio of verbal frames and visual frames, though this is, in principle, possible

Note: Subject = the person depicted.

prejudiced against methods other than their own may be diminishing (Dan, 2018, in press). Quantitatively oriented scholars are unlikely to choose, say, the hermeneutic approach or the manual holistic one to identify verbal frames, or the ideological approach to reveal visual frames.[5] Instead, they might prefer the manual-clustering approach, which promises high reliability and validity, aspects much valued in the quantitative tradition.

Moreover, I expect that, as the resources at one's disposal are always limited, (3) most scholars would have to decide between in-depth analyses or large-sample studies. Scholars confronted with large samples but who must also keep an eye on the budget are more likely to opt for the manual holistic approach or for the computer-assisted approach to identify verbal frames and for one of the denotative approaches to investigate visual frames. On the other hand, I doubt that those aiming for in-depth analyses of small samples of texts and visuals would choose any of these approaches. The alternatives listed in Table 3.2 seem more likely. Given the approaches available, scholars may have to compromise, at least when they are not open to combining various approaches.

Finally, I believe that (4) methodological triangulation (see Denzin, 2009, p. 301) may lie behind researchers' decision to identify frames through one approach or the other. In this case, scholars attempt to identify the same frames through two or more different approaches. A recent example is the study by David et al. (2011), who investigated the same sample twice, once using the manual-clustering approach and once using the manual holistic approach. They obtained similar results, leading them to believe that both approaches are equally valid (David et al., 2011). From a theory-building perspective, being able to identify the same frames using different approaches is very encouraging. It is important to note, however, that there is a possibility that different methods may produce complementary but otherwise different results (Bilandzic, 2008). Such differences would have to be addressed.

A final general remark I would like to make concerns the relationship between framing analysis and content analysis. Most approaches reviewed above collect their data by means of content analysis, suggesting that content analysis is the methodology, whereas framing is the theory. Content analysis should not be confounded with framing analysis. In my view, content analysis acts as an enabler of framing analysis. Specifically, in framing studies, content analysis is "[guided] by a framing paradigm" (Entman, 1993, p. 57). This means that scholars must explain how the constructs they identify by means of content analysis do "'organizing' and 'structuring' work" (Reese, 2007, p. 151). Where this explanation is missing, the frame status of the identified constructs is debatable.

Notes

1 Note how these reasoning devices perform the four framing functions proposed by Entman (1993): problem definition, causal interpretation, moral evaluation, and treatment recommendation.

2 In Matthes's (2009) content analysis of 131 framing articles, only 5% acknowledged visuals (see also Scheufele, 2001).

3 This resembles the way visuals were treated in the hermeneutic approach reviewed toward the beginning of this chapter.

4 Quantitative content analysis allows researchers to systematically classify observable content into categories and thus to quantify it (Bell, 2001; Krippendorff, 2013; Lutz & Collins, 1993; Rose, 2012). Guided by their respective research questions and hypotheses, scholars use content analytical methods to reduce a large amount of material to a series of codes. These codes can then be analyzed using mathematical or statistical measures (e.g., frequency analyses). Qualitative content analysis was proposed as an alternative, enabling scholars to account not just for manifest, but also for latent meaning; to pay attention to context; and to conduct analyses that were more data-driven and less focused on frequencies (Schreier, 2012). Manifest content is obvious, readily perceived, while latent content is hidden, present but not obvious (Freud, 1952). Critical methods, in turn, are concerned with "understanding the manner in which social power relationships are constituted, maintained, and perpetuated through discourse" (Kline, 2014, p. 805). These scholars "are not trying to meet the standards of objectivity, generalizability, or replicability" (Kline, 2014, p. 807).

5 I do not intend to suggest that these approaches are unreliable or invalid (see David et al., 2011; Van Gorp, 2010).

4 Factors Influencing the Act of Framing

I have argued repeatedly that framing involves the *selection* of one interpretation out of a range of alternatives and its *emphasis* in a text or in a visual. Yet, what has been unaccounted for thus far are the factors influencing these acts of selection and emphasis. In this chapter, I consider the reasons journalists and other actors convey the frames that they do.

The Context

Several authors made room for the possibility that frames are being used without ulterior motives (e.g., Gamson, 1989). From this perspective, frames in news, information subsidies, and so on are used simply to make sense of the world through the lens of prevalent ideology,[1] values and norms in the underlying culture, and political views (Berger & Luckmann, 1967; Goffman, 1974; Ryan & Gamson, 2009). These scholars believed that journalists and other social and political actors employed frames with "no motive other than a conscientious effort to frame events in a way [considered] most meaningful" (Gamson, 1989, p. 158).

While it is possible, even likely, that ideology, culture, economy, and politics would also affect advocacy frames, I could not track any studies providing empirical proof of this. However, several studies into news framing acknowledged the "societal context in which communication occurred" (Graber, 1976, p. 101), with interesting results.

Specifically, previous research suggested that the societal context affects news framing of various issues including Supreme Court decisions (Clawson, Strine, & Waltenburg, 2003), obesity (Rim, Lee, & Han, 2009), and HIV/AIDS (Bates, 2007; Krishnan, Durrah, & Winkler, 1997). More sensitive framing was found in news outlets in highly affected regions or targeted at highly affected populations. The same tendency was reported for visual coverage, though without reference to framing (Temoshok, Grade, & Zich, 1988).

Yet, as suggested in the introduction to this chapter, it is difficult to ascertain if such differences in framing are attributable to differences in the societal context alone. Prevalent ideas, norms, and values could also be used purposefully in framing in an attempt to reach specific goals (see Hallahan, 2015).

DOI: 10.4324/9781315171456-4

Interests and Goals

Previous literature explained that various actors—in full consideration of their interests and goals—carefully convey frames they then infuse in information subsidies and other culturally available messages.[2] For consistency purposes, I refer to these deliberately conveyed frames as "advocacy frames"[3] throughout this book. From this perspective, any analysis of verbal or visual frames would be incomplete without a consideration of the goals and interests of the communicator (see Halawa, 2008; Hüppauf & Weingart, 2009; Knoblauch, 2002; Lewis & Jhally, 1998; McNair, 1998; Schudson, 1991; Schwan & Zahn, 2006).

Previous research attested to the existence of advocacy frames (see Benford & Snow, 2000; Entman, 2004; Entman, Matthes, & Pellicano, 2008; Fröhlich, 2008; Gamson & Modigliani, 1987; Gandy, 2001; Hallahan, 1999, 2015; Ihlen & Nitz, 2008; Pan & Kosicki, 2001; Sheafer & Gabay, 2009; Strömbäck et al., 2013; Tewksbury, Jones, Peske, & Vig, 2000; Van Gorp, 2007; Zoller, 2014).

Scholars cautioned, however, that the goals pursued through communication may not be readily apparent (Gamson, Croteau, Hoynes, & Sasson, 1992), especially when these goals were pursued visually (Messaris, 1994, 1998). While visuals can be used deliberately (Bock, Isermann, & Knieper, 2012; Dahlgren, 2008; Emmison & Smith, 2012; Lundell, 2010; Tiemens, 1978), this is less obvious than when words are used in a similar fashion. Visuals "appear to record rather than transform and signify" (Woollacott, 1982, p. 99), which makes them seem more credible than words, closer to reality and truth (Barthes, 1981; Butler, 2007; Drew & Grimes, 1987; Joffe, 2008; Müller, 2007; Pfau et al., 2006; Ritchin, 1990; Wolf, 2008).

According to Messaris and Abraham (2001), visuals share the following three characteristics: indexicality, analogical quality, and a lack of propositional syntax. *Indexicality* means that visuals serve as "direct pointers" to what they represent. *Analogical quality* means that visuals are similar/analogous to real objects or persons and can be understood in reference to them (rather than relying on social conventions, as is necessary for words). Finally, the *lack of an explicit propositional syntax* means there are no explicit syntactic conventions for making propositions through visuals. Rather, "the conventions for making such connections are loose, imprecise, and unsystematic" (p. 218).

This makes visual advocacy frames all the more interesting for research, because the impact of framing depends on it being taken for granted, and because the framing through visuals is more likely to achieve this taken-for-granted quality than framing through words (see Messaris & Abraham, 2001).

Various actors "compete to dominate the text"—and, I would add, the visuals—of the news coverage with their advocacy frames (Entman,

1993, p. 53). In this framing contest, each actor tries to promote just one key frame—clearly distinguishable from that of the competition—per issue (Hänggli & Kriesi, 2012; Van Gorp, 2010). Communicators hoping to improve the odds that the issue at hand will be covered in a certain way increase the availability of communication carrying advocacy frames (Benford & Snow, 2000; Carragee & Roefs, 2004; Dan & Ihlen, 2011a; Gamson & Modigliani, 1989; Gandy, 1982; Hallahan, 1999; Reber & Berger, 2005)—something known as frame sponsorship (Pan & Kosicki, 2001). The purpose of frame sponsorship is to influence news framing through advocacy frames—a key component of what scholars call *frame building* (Scheufele, 1999).

Frame-Building Research

Scholars generally agree that journalists do more than just provide a "bulleted list of facts" (Sotirovic & McLeod, 2004, p. 376) like "an information bulletin board" (Bennett, 2005, p. 128). Rather, as argued by Kosicki and Pan (1997), the media can be understood "as both an agent and venue"[4] (p. 8, cited in Carragee & Roefs, 2004). Journalists have "discretionary power" over the frames transmitted to audiences (Blumler & Gurevitch, 1995, p. 87; Semetko, Blumler, Gurevitch, & Weaver, 1991, p. 3): They do not necessarily passively forward advocacy frames; they can also contrast various advocacy frames to one another or disseminate their own interpretation (Baresch, Hsu, & Reese, 2012; Bartholomé, Lecheler, & de Vreese, 2015; Brüggemann, 2014; Callaghan & Schnell, 2001; D'Angelo & Kuypers, 2010; de Vreese, 2010; Grunig, 2007; Hänggli & Kriesi, 2010; Ihlen, Figenschou, & Larsen, 2015; Johnson-Cartee, 2004; Lengauer & Höller, 2013; Nelson & Willey, 2001; Strömbäck & Esser, 2009).

Frame-building research investigates the influence of actors external to the media on the news coverage (Scheufele, 1999). Another name for this line of research includes "advanced research in determination theory" (Fröhlich, 2008) and "media agenda setting" (Dearing & Rogers, 1996). Also, in my opinion, there is great overlap between frame building and second-level agenda building (Kiousis, Mitrook, Xu, & Seltzer, 2006), although scholars in the agenda-setting tradition may see this differently.

Frame building shares characteristics with other, more popular research traditions in our discipline, especially with agenda building (Lang & Lang, 1981) and determination theory (Baerns, 1979), which can be understood as the German correspondent of agenda building. Research in agenda building and determination theory generally suggested there is a connection among the media agenda, the timing of topics, and information subsidies, respectively. Yet the strength of these connections is still unclear, mostly because of the use of different quota and yardsticks in various studies (see Donsbach & Meißner, 2004; Fröhlich & Rüdiger, 2004; Raupp, 2008).

Instead of using the media agenda and the timing of coverage as dependent variables (see Kiousis, Laskin, & Kim, 2009; Raupp, 2008), frame-building research uses media frames as the dependent variable[5] and investigates the factors that influence "the creation or changes of frames applied by journalists" (Scheufele, 1999, p. 115).

It is possible that frame-building research emerged out of what appeared to be an across-the-board dismissal of external actors' influence on news in research through the agenda-building and, especially, the determination theory perspectives. This is because frame-building scholars do not deem external influences on news as negative in and of themselves (see also Len-Ríos et al., 2009; Reich, 2006, 2009; Strömbäck & Nord, 2006). I reckon most frame-building scholars would only become suspicious when news frames matched advocacy frames to a high degree, especially when some actors advocating frames were systematically favored over others.

Previous research suggested that actors' power and resources have a lasting impact on the chances that their advocacy frames will be picked up by journalists (Arroyave, 2012; Carragee & Roefs, 2004; Corbett & Mori, 1999; Entman, 1993, 2004; Reese, 2001; Sheafer & Gabay, 2009). This recalls the indexing hypothesis, which stated that "mass media news professionals ... tend to 'index' the range of voices and viewpoints ... according to the range of views expressed in mainstream government debate about a given topic" (Bennett, 1990, p. 106).

In Lawrence's (2010) words, "the indexing hypothesis speaks directly to the question of news framing" (p. 269; see also Hänggli, 2012). In his cascading activation model, Entman (2003) modeled the way the indexing hypothesis "speaks" to framing. In a later publication, Entman (2004) argued that frames originating from the administration/elites flow to the bottom—that is, to the media and then to the public.

When powerful and resourceful actors "have ideological inertia on their side" (Ryan, 1991, p. 68), the reproduction of their advocacy frames in the news would solidify existing power relations, making social change more difficult (Arroyave, 2012; Gramsci, 1971; Lupton, 1994c). Critical scholars speak here of hegemony (Kline, 2014; Spinetta, 2014; Turow & Coe, 1993). Critical scholars also investigate whose interests are being served by visuals (Pieterse, 1992) or, in a more general sense, whose interpretation visuals privilege (Hall, 1997). These scholars often conclude that dominant groups use visuals to establish and maintain hegemonic power (Hariman & Lucaites, 2007; Jewitt, 2008; Tagg, 1988). For instance, scholars suggest that the visuals used in the reporting of military conflict (Fahmy, 2004a; Griffin, 2004; Moriarty & Show, 1995; Reynolds & Barnett, 2003) and crime (Barnett, 2003; Fahmy, Bock, & Wanta, 2014; Finn, 2009; Howe, 2006; Messaris & Abraham, 2001) maintain the organization of social reality in the way preferred by dominant groups. Thus, visuals are "very effective tools for framing and articulating ideological messages" (Messaris & Abraham, 2001, p. 220), which makes visual framing "a prime site of ideological constructions expressed within news stories" (Coleman, 2010, p. 238).

Yet other factors may also affect journalistic decisions to pass on frames to audiences. Knowledge about how framing works, especially, and skills in conveying advocacy frames can increase the likelihood that they are picked up (see Pan & Kosicki, 2001; Ryan, 1991). In an earlier publication, we provided an overview of these skills, which we named "framing expertise" (see Dan & Ihlen, 2011a).

To summarize, extrapolating from Maat and de Jong (2013), the question for frame-building scholars is not *whether* journalists use culturally available messages and information subsidies or not, but *how* they use them (p. 350, original emphasis). A similar line of reasoning was advanced by Williams and Miller (1995).

Despite frequent calls for research into "the conditions under which [news] frames emerge" (de Vreese, 2005, p. 60),[6] very few researchers have responded with an investigation of frame building. Reese (2007) cautioned that current scholarship runs the risk of "reifying [frames]—locking them in place, as though they were not part of a larger conversation, serving particular interests, and undergoing changes over time" (p. 149).

Borah's (2011) content analysis of published framing research testified to the severity of this research gap: Only 2.3% of 379 recent framing studies investigated frame building (Borah, 2011). This gap is especially noticeable for visual frame building, which was described as "greatly underdocumented" (Grabe & Bucy, 2009, p. 129). In a recent systematic review of 29 studies of visual framing, the authors found that only one study researched visual frames from a communicator perspective (Geise, Lobinger, & Brantner, 2013).

Despite the low number of studies, two main paths to frame-building research could be identified—they are reviewed below in more depth. One group of scholars investigated the connection between news source prevalence and news frames; the other determined the extent to which advocacy frames resemble news frames. This latter research avenue appears to have emerged out of the difficulties inherent to research projects linking news sources to news frames. As journalists do not always reveal their sources (Raupp, 2014; Swain, 2007; Tanner & Friedman, 2011), a "smokescreen of anonymity" emerges (Reich, 2010, p. 811), complicating such research projects. Yet, irrespective of which of these two research avenues they pursued, scholars did not offer their results as evidence of causal relationships between advocacy frames and news frames. Instead, they cautiously pointed to a link between the two without making claims of causality.

Recently, a third strategy in frame-building research was proposed by Boesman, d'Haenens, and Van Gorp (2016). These authors outlined an ethnographic model combining content analysis with ethnography across four phases of research, namely (1) newsroom observations, (2) news frame analysis, (3) reconstruction interviews, and (4) frame-building analysis. It is too early to judge if this strategy will catch on, but its potential is very high. Should it win wide recognition, then a third path to frame-building research will emerge.

News Source Prevalence and News Frames

Journalists and news sources need one another and benefit from one another[7] (Brandenburg, 2002; Gandy, 1982; Shoemaker, 1991; Sigal, 1986; Turk, 1985). Yet too much closeness may reduce journalists to being mouthpieces.

One group of scholars investigating frame building attempted to find out whether or not the prevalence of certain news sources in a story affected media framing. From sourcing studies in general, we know that powerful and elite actors are often favored as news sources (Andsager & Smiley, 1998; Berkowitz, 1987; Berres, 2014; Coleman, 1995; Corbett & Mori, 1999; Gans, 1980; Hänggli, 2012; Hornig-Priest & Talbert, 1994; Raupp, 2008; Schudson, 2003, 2006; Sigal, 1973; Tanner & Friedman, 2011; Williams & Miller, 1995). For instance, the police were clearly favored over other sources in stories about law violation (see O'Neill & O'Connor, 2008; Pollack & Allern, 2014), especially on local news (Trautman, 2004). Recently, Bock and Araiza (2015) showed that law enforcement institutions acting as sources had great power over news framing.

Previous research showed that newsrooms tend to rely on a limited number of sources (Baerns, 1991; Berkowitz, 1991), and the information provided to journalists by external actors affects their coverage (Adoni & Mane, 1984; Arroyave, 2012; Berkowitz & Adams, 1990; Carter, Stamm, & Heintz-Knowles, 1992; Coleman, 1995; Donohue, Tichenor, & Olien, 1973; Durham, 1998; Salwen, 1995; Stocking, 1985; Strömbäck et al., 2013; Weaver & Elliott, 1986).

According to previous frame-building research, there appears to be a connection between the use of certain news sources and media frames (Coleman, 1995; D'Angelo & Kuypers, 2010; Dimitrova & Strömbäck, 2012; Strömbäck et al., 2013; Tankard, 2001). The number of studies taking this innovative approach to frame building is quite low, however, so it is unclear whether journalists' systematic favoring of some sources over others has a lasting effect on news framing. This would be particularly problematic in the case of single-sourced news accounts, where one source would assume the entire power over news framing.

This line of reasoning may well apply to visual frames, in that the use of certain photo sources may be associated with the use of certain visual news frames. To my knowledge, no study to date has investigated this.

Link between Advocacy Frames and News Frames

Another group of scholars compared news frames to advocacy frames in information subsidies and culturally available messages, such as news releases, political ads, and interviews (Bedingfield & Anshari, 2014; Hänggli & Kriesi, 2012; Raupp, 2014). While news releases were often scrutinized in such research projects, some scholars argued in favor of expanding the focus to other types of information carrying advocacy frames (see Reich, 2010).

Current research results paint a mixed picture. Callaghan and Schnell (2001) discovered a "systematic link" between advocacy frames and news frames in the media coverage of gun control legislation (p. 201). Another study also concluded that news frames were "remarkably similar" to advocacy frames in the media coverage of physician-assisted suicide (Holody, 2009, p. 20). Several other investigations obtained comparable results (Andsager & Smiley, 1998; Powers & Andsager, 1999; Raupp, 2014; Rim et al., 2009; Weissman, 2014). Yet at least three studies suggested that news frames were richer than advocacy frames (Lee, 2014; Lee & Basnyat, 2012; Nucci, Cuite, & Hallman, 2009).

All the studies mentioned in the paragraph above focused on verbal frames. To my knowledge, the only study analyzing visual frame building is Grabe and Bucy's (2009). These authors compared TV news coverage with the image construction strategies of image handlers working for presidential candidates. Grabe and Bucy (2009) explained how the images of political candidates were "constructed visually through deliberate campaign strategies designed to promote desired qualities and favorite themes" (p. 85). They discovered many similarities between the "visual frames orchestrated by image handlers" for political candidates and visual news frames (Grabe & Bucy, 2009, p. 128).

Notes

1 An ideology is "a set of general beliefs or abstract values by which people define the social and political arrangements that they believe ought to be preferred" (Kay & Eibach, 2012, p. 496).

2 Gandy (1982) coined the term "information subsidies" to denote the information provided by external actors to journalists, such as news releases and backgrounders (p. 61). "Culturally available" messages, on the other hand, is a broader term encompassing all types of purposeful communication that may influence journalists, regardless of whether it was addressed to them or not (Gamson & Modigliani, 1987, p. 144).

3 Note, however, that these frames are encountered in the literature under various names, including strategic, actor, and advocacy frames (Brüggemann, 2014; de Vreese, 2010; Hallahan, 2008).

4 Similarly, Callaghan and Schnell (2001) spoke of a "dual role of the media" (p. 186), while Pan and Kosicki (1993) described media's role as "active" (p. 55). News stories are a venue for framing contests, "providing a clean canvas upon which contenders painted their claims" (Coleman, 1995, p. 72).

5 In principle, frame-building research can investigate three sources of influence on news framing: sponsoring activities, ideology, and organizational pressures (Bennett, Lawrence, & Livingston, 2006; de Vreese, 2003, 2005; Dimitrova & Kostadinova, 2013; Hänggli & Kriesi, 2010; Scheufele, 1999, 2000; Tedesco, 2001; Zhou & Moy, 2007). In empirical studies, however, frame building has often been limited to how advocacy frames in information subsidies and culturally available messages influence news frames; a notable exception is Dimitrova and Kostadinova's (2013) study.

6 Similar statements can be encountered in many publications (e.g., Carragee & Roefs, 2004; de Vreese & Lecheler, 2012; Entman et al., 2008; Müller, 2013; Pan & Kosicki, 2001; Wise & Brewer, 2010).

7 Bentele, Liebert, and Seeling (1997) tried to model this complex relationship under the rubric *intereffication approach* (see for details Wehmeier, 2008). The authors describe the relationship between actors external to news media and their information subsidies on the one hand and journalism on the other hand as one of mutual influence, orientation, and dependence. By sharing their information and views with journalists—by becoming news sources—social and political actors have the opportunity to reach large audiences and policymakers. Their dependence on journalism is obvious. Conversely, journalists need the information provided by social and political actors to produce news, thus to get access to information and to confer legitimacy to a newscast (Coleman, 1995; Conrad, 1999; Kim & Weaver, 2003; Len-Ríos et al., 2009; Tanner, 2004). For instance, journalists may "speak" through their sources, which they carefully choose to make the argument they wanted to make in the first place but lacked legitimacy. The line of research investigating this phenomenon conceptualizes news sources as "opportune witnesses" (Hagen, 1993, p. 317).

5 An Introduction to Integrative Framing Analysis

The literature reviewed in Chapter 2 advanced several arguments in favor of integrative framing analyses. One was that, as most messages consist of both words and visuals, analyzing just the words or just the visuals in a given message is inevitably incomplete. Previous studies also suggested that visuals attract attention better than words, stand better chances to be processed ahead of and faster than words, and are remembered better. Yet, as argued above, using these results to justify focusing on the visual channel of communication alone seems equally inadequate. When a message consists of words and visuals, the sensible thing to do is to analyze both channels of communication. The value of integrative framing studies is beyond dispute, especially when the words and visuals convey conflicting frames, as audiences are likely to retain the visual interpretation over the verbal interpretation. Integrative framing analyses can highlight how much meaning gets lost in studies focusing on just one channel of communication (see Chapter 2).

Calls for framing analyses that pay attention to both words and visuals are justified (Coleman, 2010; Lobinger & Geise, 2013), but the number of framing studies analyzing both words and visuals is quite small (see Chapter 3). An exploration into why this is the case was undertaken in Chapter 3. Based on the literature reviewed there, I argue the reason lies in the paucity of methodological guidance regarding data collection and data analysis in integrative studies. If up until recently scholars ignored visuals in framing studies because of methodological difficulties, it is possible that history is repeating itself with integrative framing studies. The question now is not how to analyze verbal frames or visual frames, as advice is widely available in this regard (see Chapter 3). Rather, the question is, *How can integrative framing analyses be conducted?*

The purpose of this chapter is to provide a detailed and hands-on answer to this question, in an effort to assist scholars attempting to conduct integrative framing analyses. In Chapter 6, my approach is put to a test; the empirical study shows precisely what each of the proposed steps looks like in practice.

DOI: 10.4324/9781315171456-5

Chapter 3 ended with my appraisal of the current approaches to integrative framing analyses. There, I clearly stated my preference for collecting the verbal and visual data separately before reconnecting the two data sets during data analysis. Here, I argue that, although it may seem counterintuitive, conducting an integrative framing analysis means conducting two separate analyses—one verbal, one visual (Coleman, 2010). Separating the words from the visuals during data collection is a prerequisite to integrating them during data analysis. This is essential if scholars want to prevent obscuring much of the meaning visuals convey independently from words and vice versa, especially when the messages conveyed by the two channels of communication conflict.[1]

Figure 5.1 contains a flowchart of the process of integrative framing analysis, with six steps outlined. Many of the steps displayed parallel those of other types of research (e.g., codebook development and data collection). The distinctive feature of this approach is that four of the six steps are carried out separately for words and visuals, as denoted by labels such as "Step 2a" and "Step 2b," where "a" stands for performing the step in the verbal sample and "b" for the visual sample. As suggested by the block arrows at the bottom of Figure 5.1, the first three steps relate to the preparation of the material for the analysis and to the preparation of the analysis. The fourth step involves the data collection; the fifth and sixth steps concern the data analysis. In the remainder of this chapter, I account for each of the steps in detail, referring back to this visualization.

Preparation

As shown in Figure 5.1, three steps are necessary to prepare for an integrative framing analysis. The first step involves disjoining words from visuals in the sample and is a prerequisite for the next steps. The second step is to select a verbal and a visual approach to identify verbal and visual frames, respectively. The third step involves developing two research instruments, one for the words and one for the visuals.

Step 1: Separation of Words and Visuals

The first step is administrative and can be delegated to research assistants. It entails separating words from visuals (see Figure 5.1) for each item in the sample—for each news article, for example. Prior to the separation, an identification number should be assigned to each item. For instance, the first news article consisting of both words and visuals should be given the identification number "1."

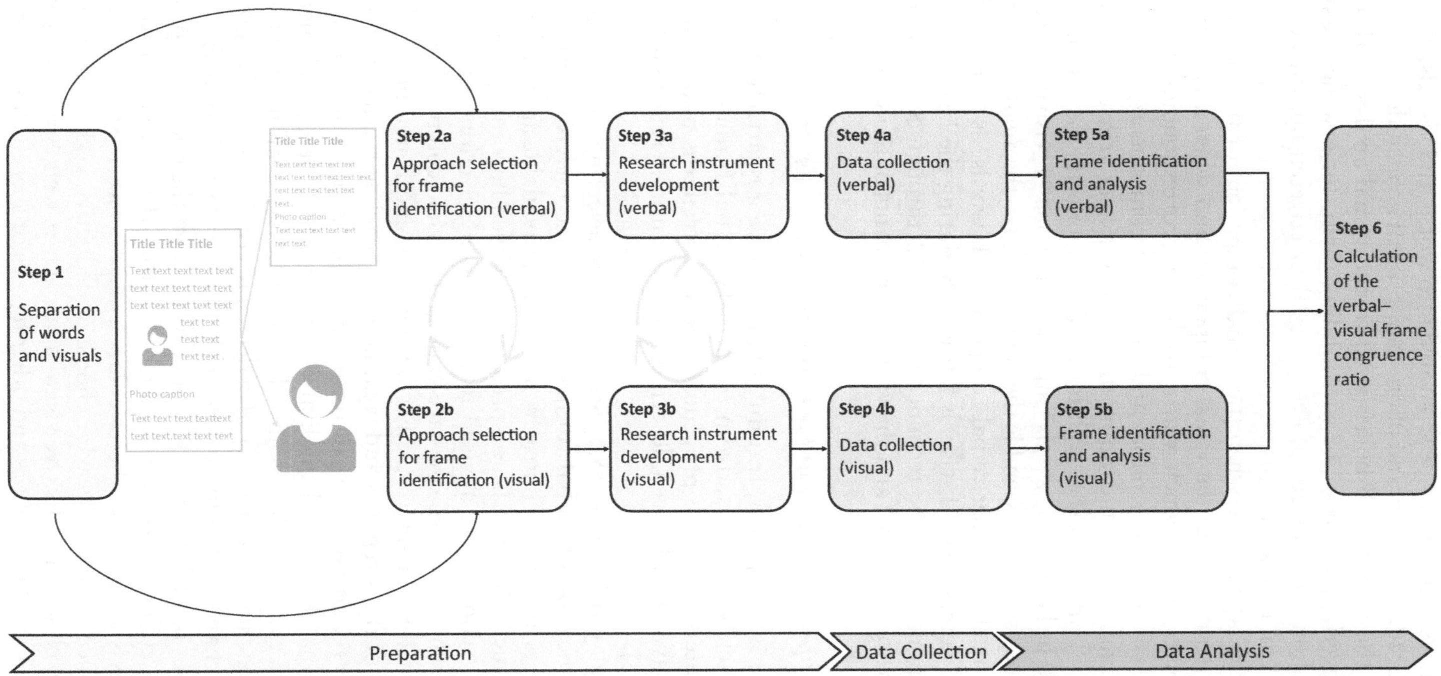

Figure 5.1 Step-by-Step Process for Integrative Framing Analysis.

Each news article must be separated into words and visuals. The headline, subhead, text body, and photo caption will be included in the verbal analysis; the visuals will be assigned to the visual analysis. All text in visuals, overlapping them, or surrounding them (for instance, text on a banner) should be cut out of every visual or covered up. Image editing software can be used to this end.

This step is complete when the verbal component of the sample is archived separately from the visual component, and when it is clear which visuals correspond to which words. To this end, corresponding ID numbers must be assigned to the verbal and the visual components of each material. For example, when dividing the first newspaper article in the sample ("article 1") into its verbal and its visual components, the verbal component could be labeled "1_words" and the visual one "1_visuals." These IDs can then be used to re-assemble the news article for the analysis (Step 6), as the labeling clarifies that verbal component "1_words" is associated with the visual component "1_visuals." It is only during the last step that the two components will be reconnected. Steps 2 through 5 are performed separately for the verbal and the visual components of the sample.

Step 2: Approach Selection for Frame Identification

As shown in Chapter 3, framing scholars have a relatively wide range of approaches to choose from to identify verbal frames and their visual counterparts. The procedure and the strengths and weaknesses of each have already been described and will not be repeated here (see Chapter 3).

As displayed in Figure 5.1, Step 2 entails selecting an approach for the identification of verbal frames (2a) and one for visual frames (2b). Researchers are free to choose from any of the available approaches those that best meet their needs and preferences. Given how many approaches there are, scholars are advised to justify their selection and to specify how and why the approaches are expected to yield comparable data.

As argued in Chapter 3, this choice may be motivated not just by an appraisal of the strengths and weaknesses of each approach, but also by researchers' understanding of frames as either generic or issue-specific; their inclination toward qualitative, quantitative, or critical methods; the resources at their disposal; and, possibly, by an aspiration to triangulate approaches. Scholars may also decide to combine several approaches for each channel of communication (verbal or visual) to attenuate the weaknesses of each approach. It's important that the selected approaches allow the collection of comparable data from the words and from the visuals, as suggested by the circular arrows between Steps 2a and 2b. For instance, researchers who choose a deductive verbal approach are advised to choose a deductive visual approach as well. Similarly, scholars analyzing verbal metaphors and other figures of speech should also code visual metaphors, symbols, and so on.

The approach to integrative framing analysis proposed in this chapter works, in principle, with frames identified through each of the approaches reviewed in Chapter 3, as long as the frames are identified separately for each channel.

This step is complete when researchers have decided on at least one approach to identify verbal frames and at least one to identify visual frames.

Step 3: Research Instrument Development

Developing the research instrument is the last step in preparing for an integrative framing analysis. The researcher must now determine how the data will be collected. This decision depends on the nature of the sample selected for analysis and on whether the researcher prefers quantitative, qualitative, or critical methods. It affects the flexibility of the data collection, the amount of detail provided in the research instrument, and the decision to collect data personally or to delegate it to research assistants. As a general remark, I advise against using holistic measures when researchers analyze material from contexts with which they are not very familiar (e.g., foreign country, foreign language, etc.).

High-quality advice on quantitative and qualitative content analysis and on critical studies is widely available elsewhere and will not be repeated here (see, e.g., Krippendorff, 2013; Ott & Mack, 2014; Schreier, 2012). Regardless of one's methodological preferences, the development of the research instrument should be guided by the research questions and, where applicable, the hypotheses the researcher wishes to address. For qualitative and quantitative studies, the goal is to determine which characteristics of the texts and visuals in the sample are of interest and how they can be turned into variables that can be observed and recorded. To this end, these variables must be operationally defined.

Next, the researcher undertakes the task of developing two separate but corresponding research instruments, one for words and one for visuals. This step is, perhaps, the most difficult in integrative framing analysis.

The two research instruments are interconnected, and their development becomes an iterative and interactive process, as denoted by the circular arrows between Steps 3a and 3b in Figure 5.1. For instance, a researcher beginning with the development of the research instrument for the words has already decided which variables are of interest and how they can be captured when expressed verbally. The next task is to determine how, if at all, the visual expression of these variables can be operationalized. Here it is necessary to constantly compare the two research instruments to determine a verbal and a visual expression of each aspect of interest.

This step is a sensitive one, as researchers new to visual research may be tempted to try to capture the meaning conveyed by visuals in a way that does not do justice to the differences between words and visuals (see Chapter 2). It is crucial that the researchers not attempt to simply cast the verbal research instrument into a visual mold, forcing visual meaning into categories derived verbally. Instead, scholars must constantly ask themselves if the way they intend to capture visual meaning leads to the desired results.

At this stage, researchers should also determine the type of meaning they are interested in and the unit of analysis. They might be interested in either manifest or latent meaning. The unit of analysis might be an entire piece of material (say, the words in a news article or the photo in that article) or a specific issue or individual—depending on the type of framing scholars are interested in.

When two research instruments exist, Step 3 is complete. These instruments should help the researchers to capture aspects of the verbal and visual dimensions of interest. Before data collection can begin in the next step, scholars should ensure through sufficient training that they or the assistants they entrust with the data collection have a very good command of the research instruments. Also, this is the stage when they, especially those using quantitative methods, should run pretests and tests for reliability.

Data Collection

Step 4: Data Collection

Step 4 is concerned with data collection from the verbal and visual components of the sample, respectively. As shown in Figure 5.1, unlike the procedure for Steps 2 and 3, Steps 4a and 4b are independent of each other. In the figure, this is signaled by the absence of circular arrows between the verbal and the visual stages of the step.

Researchers should try to prevent any amalgamation of the data collected from the verbal and visual components. In other words, researchers should make all reasonable effort to ensure that those collecting data from one channel of communication are not influenced by the meanings conveyed through the other channel of communication.

Several precautions are in order. First, the complete collection of data from one channel of communication can precede the collection of data from the other channel. Second, when data collection is delegated to research assistants, different individuals or teams can be used for each channel of communication. Third, the verbal counterpart of the visuals in one assistant's/team's subsample can be assigned to the subsample given to the other assistant/team, and vice versa.

This step is complete when two separate data sets emerge: one providing information relevant to visual framing and the other to verbal framing.

Data Analysis

The last stage in the process of integrative framing analysis—data analysis—is accomplished in Steps 5 and 6. See the last block arrow at the bottom of Figure 5.1. Here, the researcher begins the analysis of the collected data based on the objectives of the study. To this end, he or she will have to choose fitting statistical or other techniques.

Step 5: Frame Identification

In this step, the researcher identifies verbal frames and visual frames in the data collected. As suggested in Figure 5.1 by the absence of circular arrows between Steps 5a and 5b, the identification of frames is carried out separately for each channel of communication.

This step is inapplicable to studies where holistic measures are used, as the data collected are synonymous with the frames (see Chapter 3). It also may not apply to some critical and qualitative studies. But in quantitative studies where frames have been broken down into several components for data collection, scholars must now decide on a technique to merge the various components to reveal the frames. When small samples are investigated, researchers can try to do this manually. But when researchers examine large samples, it is necessary to use statistical techniques. In this case, depending on the unit of analysis and on their interest in all frames or in just the dominant one, scholars can choose between procedures such as index building, homogeneity analysis (Van Gorp, 2005), factor analysis (Semetko & Valkenburg, 2000), or cluster analysis (Matthes & Kohring, 2008), or they can opt for a combination thereof.

In keeping with Entman (1993), the task here is not just to identify the frames but also to determine how salient they are in the text or in the visual analyzed. This involves ascertaining the weight of each appearing frame (Van Gorp, 2010) by comparison to the others. In qualitative and critical studies, this may be done manually, for example by counting or by assigning varying weight to different cues. In quantitative studies, researchers can build indexes by adding up all frame elements in one variable, provided high Cronbach's alphas. The assumption is that the higher the weight of a frame, the higher is the chance that the verbal or visual message will call to the mind of the recipient a schema that is consistent with that frame (Entman, 1993; Van Gorp, 2010).

This step is complete when the researcher has identified a corpus of verbal frames and one of visual frames, respectively, and when she or he has determined each frame's salience in every text and visual.

Step 6: Calculation of the Verbal-Visual Frame Congruence Ratio

In Step 6, the words and visuals that were disjoined in Step 1 are now virtually reconnected (see Figure 5.1). This allows the researcher to calculate the verbal-visual frame congruence ratio.

In studies using qualitative and critical measures or in studies using small samples, researchers can attempt to compare the visual frames to the verbal frames for each unit of analysis manually. In quantitative studies, however, scholars need to merge the verbal and visual data sets. In doing so, choosing a long format in a statistical program or in a spreadsheet program is advisable. Each line in the data set should contain the data relevant to both the verbal and the visual frames of any given item (a news article, for example). To prevent entering the data in the wrong row by mistake, researchers should try to do this automatically. When this is not possible, the researcher must resort to the corresponding identification numbers assigned to the verbal and the visual components of each material in the sample (see Step 1). Specifically, he or she would have to allocate the first columns in the combined data set to the ID numbers for the visual and verbal components of each item. These IDs should be compared and the data import double-checked when the two IDs do not match.

Once the data collected from words and visuals are in one place, the researcher can proceed with the comparison of the verbal and visual frames. The goal here is to determine the extent to which verbal frames and visual frames reinforced or contradicted each other in the sample, something I call the verbal-visual frame congruence ratio (CR_{Frames}).

For quantitative studies, I recommend that scholars calculate this ratio for each unit of analysis by dividing the number of times the verbal frame was matched by a visual frame ($Pairs_{=}$) by the total number of visual frames ($\Sigma_{Visual\ Frames}$), as in the following formula:

$$CR_{Frames} = \frac{Pairs_{=}}{\sum_{Visual\ Frames}}$$

where CR_{Frames} is the verbal-visual frame congruence ratio; $Pairs_{=}$ is the number of frame pairs (i.e., same verbal frame and visual frame for that issue or person); and $\Sigma_{Visual\ Frames}$ is the total number of visual frames.

This means that to calculate the congruence ratio for each unit of analysis, scholars must first compute a variable recording how many visual frames were conveyed for every verbal frame[2] ($\Sigma_{Visual\ Frames}$) and a variable recording how many photos used the same frame used in the text ($Pairs_{=}$). For this formula to work, the verbal and the visual units of analysis must be comparable (e.g., verbal frames in the entire text of a news article vs. visual frames in the accompanying photos of that article).

Table 5.1 Congruence Ratio—Calculation Examples

		Visual Frame in …			*Computed Variables*		
Unit of Analysis	*Verbal Frame*	*Photo 1*	*Photo 2*	*Photo 3*	*Total number of visual frames* ($\Sigma_{Visual\ Frames}$)	*Number of pairs* ($Pairs_{=}$)	*Verbal-visual frame congruence ratio* (CR_{Frames})
1	Frame A	Frame B	Frame B	Frame B	3	0	0.00
2	Frame A	Frame A	Frame B		2	1	0.50
3	Frame A	Frame A	Frame A	Frame B	3	2	0.67
4	Frame A	Frame A	Frame A	Frame A	3	3	1.00
5	Frame A	Frame A	—*		1	1	1.00

* When the frame conveyed verbally is reinforced visually in one photo, but not in the second photo—because the second photo conveys no frame at all—SPSS should be instructed to set the congruence ratio at "1.00" nonetheless (perfect congruence). This is justified as follows: As verbal and visual congruence was fully established between the communication channels that conveyed a frame, it is unlikely that a frameless photo would weaken the impression already conveyed by the congruent verbal and visual frames.

A hypothetical example should help illustrate the above formula. Let's assume that the congruence ratio has been calculated for a news article in which one verbal frame is conveyed in the text and two visual frames are conveyed in the accompanying photos. In this case, the value "2" would be recorded in the newly created variable called $\Sigma_{\text{Visual Frames}}$.

Let's assume further that one of the photos in this article conveys the same frame that was conveyed in the text, whereas the second photo conveys a different frame. This means the verbal frame was reinforced in just one of the two photos. In this case, the value "1" must be recorded in SPSS in the newly computed variable $\text{Pairs}_{=}$.

The congruence ratio would then be calculated by dividing 1 (which was the number of frame pairs) by 2 (which was the total number of visual frames). The congruence ratio would thus be 0.50 or 50%. Table 5.1 includes several other calculation examples.

$$CR_{\text{Frames}} = \frac{\text{Pairs}_{=}}{\sum_{\text{Visual Frames}}} = \frac{1}{2} = 0.50$$

A prerequisite for calculating a verbal-visual frame congruence ratio for news article or other type of communication is that it consists of both words and visuals that can be compared to each other. The ratio cannot be calculated when that message consists of just words or just visuals (e.g., a newspaper article without photos). Similarly, a congruence ratio cannot be calculated when only a verbal or only a visual frame was identified in that message. A summary is offered in Table 5.2.

With the completion of this step, the integrative framing analysis is finalized and the researcher can move to the discussion of the results in light of the theory and previous empirical studies.

Table 5.2 Circumstances under which the Congruence Ratio cannot be Calculated

Frames			*Circumstances*				
Unit of Analysis	*Verbal*	*Visual*	*#1: No Frame*	*#2: Only Verbal Message*	*#3: Only Visual Message*	*#4: Only Verbal Frame*	*#5: Only Visual Frame*
1	No frame	No frame	✓				
2	Frame A	No photo		✓			
3	No text	Frame A			✓		
4	Frame A	No frame				✓	
5	No frame	Frame A					✓

Notes

1 As Parry (2010) put it, an image can "reinforce" or "undermine" the frame in a text; see Chapter 2.

2 This must not be confounded with the total number of photos, as it is possible that the total number of visual frames will differ from the total number of photos.

For instance, a news article illustrated with three photos can convey up to three visual frames (one in each photo). But when only two of the photos convey a frame and the third does not, the number of visual frames is lower than the number of photos.

6 An Integrative Framing Analysis of People Living with HIV/AIDS

The purpose of this chapter is to demonstrate the approach to integrative framing analysis proposed in Chapter 5. To this end, an analysis of the verbal frames, the visual frames, and the interplay between verbal and visual frames conveyed for people living with HIV/AIDS (PLWHA) is presented. The sample was drawn from news, special interest and niche publications (SIPs), and public service announcements (PSAs). The investigation also considers verbal and visual frame building (see Chapter 4).

In the section "Literature Review," I offer a brief review of how prevalent ideas, norms, and values have been applied to HIV/AIDS during the 35 years since its emergence. In the second part, I turn to the four frames of interest in this study, namely the normal, carrier, survivor, and victim frames. In "Research Questions, Hypotheses, and Strategy of Analysis," I present the assumptions that will be tested in this study and an overview of the statistical procedures used in the data analysis. In "Methodology," I describe the sample and the sampling procedure, justify my selection of approaches for the identification of verbal and visual frames, and describe the codebooks and the coding process. "Results" is devoted to the presentation of the findings. Here I present the frames and their components, and address the hypotheses and research questions. In "Discussion," I turn to what each of the findings means for communication scholarship and practice.

Literature Review

Prevalent Ideologies and HIV/AIDS in the United States

At the time of this study, HIV/AIDS had been around for about 35 years and remained incurable. A dramatic upsurge in deaths from HIV/AIDS was projected by 2030 (Mathers & Loncar, 2006). However, treatment that increased the chances that PLWHA would live long and fruitful lives was available (CDC, 2015b). This means that HIV/AIDS remains an incurable disease; yet, it became manageable.

DOI: 10.4324/9781315171456-6

Compared to other health problems, HIV/AIDS affects a relatively low percentage of Americans (CDC, 2013b). About 1.2 million Americans currently live with HIV, most of them men (76%). In 2010, gay and bisexual men accounted for 78% of new infections among men. By race and ethnicity, blacks/African Americans and Hispanics/Latinos are disproportionately affected by HIV. Overall, more than 650,000 people with an AIDS diagnosis have died in the United States (CDC, 2013b).

Accordingly, HIV/AIDS can be considered an "unobtrusive" medical condition, meaning that most people's thoughts and feelings about HIV/AIDS do not rest on direct experience (Nelkin, 1987, p. 63). Rather, people are likely to encounter this topic mostly in news accounts, public health campaigns, advertising, and other types of communication. For most people, then, mass distributed messages about HIV/AIDS function as a window to a world not experienced firsthand[1] (see Bennett, 2005; Bird & Dardenne, 1988; Elliott, 2011; Patterson, 1994). HIV/AIDS may be particularly prone to social construction through verbal and visual communication. Social construction means that what we know, feel, and think about diseases and those living with them is shaped by our culture, media diets, and the communication of powerful actors (Bohan, 1996; Dutta, 2014; Lupton, 2000; Maddux & Lopez, 2015; McAllister, 1992; Rosenblum & Travis, 1996; Treichler, 1988b). The language and visuals employed with reference to a certain disease socially construct that disease—much more so than biomedical and epidemiological information (see Zoller, 2014).

During the 35 years since the first confirmed case of what would later be known as AIDS, a shift has occurred in the way prevailing ideas, worldviews, and norms were brought to bear on the issue. This section shows which of the prevalent ideologies in US culture played a key role in this regard and how they were applied to the issue (Bardhan, 2002; see also Grover, 1992; Rogers, Dearing, & Chang, 1991; amfAR, 2011; Treichler, 1988a). Additionally, some key events[2] that may have led to this shift are presented. Figure 6.1 summarizes this evolution.

The first cultural elements applied to the HIV/AIDS epidemic were ethical principles and religious tenets in line with "The New Right" and "The Religious Right" (see Highleyman & Shepard, 2015). Indeed, the first confirmed case of HIV/AIDS in 1981 reached the US in the middle of a cultural shift away from the permissiveness of the 1960s and 1970s. Scholars referred to this period as one characterized by a "moral crusade" meant to promote the nuclear family, fidelity, and chastity (Highleyman & Shepard, 2015, p. 854).

At that time, the characteristics of the first people diagnosed with HIV/AIDS—gay men from large metropolitan areas like New York City and San Francisco (CDC, 1981)—served as grist for the mill of the moral crusaders. This led to the (wrongful) belief that HIV/AIDS was caused by homosexual intercourse and the "sins" of urban life—a belief that aligns well with the Bible tale of Sodom and Gomorrah

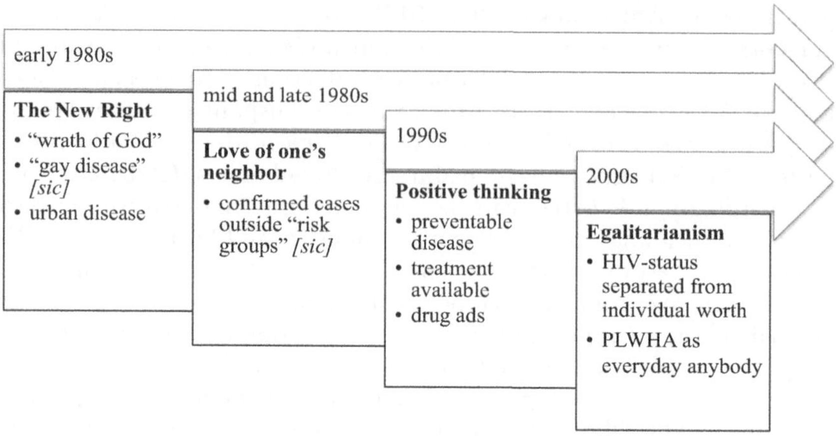

Figure 6.1 Prevalent Ideologies and HIV/AIDS in the United States.

(see Devine, Plant, & Harrison, 1999; Grover, 1992; Lupton, 1994a). HIV/AIDS was soon constructed as a punishment for a perceived decline of moral standards, as the wrath of God on those challenging prevailing norms (Albert, 1986; Baker, 1986; Campbell, Foulis, Maimane, & Sibiya, 2005; Crimp, 1988; Glick, 2011; Herek, 1999; Lupton, 1994a; McAllister, 1992; Muturi & An, 2010; Park, 1993; Sontag, 1989). This phenomenon is not new; diseases have a long history of being exploited in this way (Watney, 1988; Weeks, 1988).

At the time, mainstream media coverage of HIV/AIDS was rare, characterized by fear, and confined to guilty "risk groups" *[sic]* (Bardhan, 2002; Hertog, Finnegan, & Kahn, 1994; Kinsella, 1989). People living with HIV/AIDS were largely invisible. The only visuals were photos of body parts with grotesque lesions and microscopic views of affected tissue (Grover, 1992). This type of coverage was considered to have constructed HIV/AIDS as a self-inflicted "gay disease" and as a "gay problem" (Watney, 1990a).

In this way, the media established, reproduced, and legitimized the dominant ideology at the time (see Arroyave, 2012; Bardhan, 2001; Corbett & Mori, 1999; Fairclough, 1995; Gerbner, Gross, Morgan, & Signorielli, 1994; Herman & Chomsky, 2002; Johnson-Cartee, 2004; Kline, 2014; McCoy, 1993; Shoemaker & Reese, 1996). By pointing to dominant ideologies (Kay & Eibach, 2012), media frames seem natural and obvious (Arroyave, 2012; Berger, 1995; Hazelton, 1997; Herman & Chomsky, 2002; Hertog & McLeod, 2001; Schiller, 1973; Van Gorp, 2007, 2010). Generally speaking, people learn through the media which lifestyles to value and what counts as appropriate behavior (Bennett, 2005; Elliott, 2011; Shoemaker & Reese, 2014; Viswanath, 2006).

While the "moral crusade" went on for two full decades (Highleyman & Shepard, 2015), during the mid- and late-1980s the HIV/AIDS epidemic slowly began to be seen through an alternative cultural lens, namely, that of "love one's neighbor," a religious value subsumed to the virtue of charity. Yet, not every "neighbor" with an HIV/AIDS diagnosis experienced the same amount of love. Rather, people began to distinguish between "guilty" and "innocent" PLWHA, based on the way they had contracted the virus (Juhasz, 1990; Sacks, 1996). Children, hemophiliacs, and married men and women were generally considered innocent, while drug users, gay men, and commercial sex workers were deemed guilty. As shown in Figure 6.1, some Americans continued to apply the cultural values promoted by The New Right to PLWHA, but the tenet of "love one's neighbor" emerged as an alternative.

Two turning points occurred in 1985, namely, the diagnosis and death of Rock Hudson, a famous actor thought to be heterosexual, and the debarment from school of Ryan White, a 13-year-old boy who had contracted the virus through contaminated blood products (see Grover, 1992). Afterward, heterosexuals began to feel vulnerable to a disease (Sturken, 1997) that was sometimes constructed as having been "leaked" by a guilty minority to an innocent population (Sontag, 1989; Wellings, 1988; Williams & Miller, 1995).

Following these events, the media coverage of HIV/AIDS tripled (Albert, 1989; Nelkin, 1991; Netter, 1992; PSRA, 1996). The disease was granted "front page" status (Gross, 1991) and was no longer confined to alternative newspapers and publications intended only for a homosexual audience (Biddle, Conte, & Diamond, 1993; Rogers et al., 1991). Also, the public discourse became more sympathetic (McAllister, 1992; Sturken, 1997). In 1986, amfAR issued the first public service announcement on HIV/AIDS prevention. The Centers for Disease Control and Prevention (CDC) started a campaign called "America Responds to AIDS" the following year (amfAR, 2011).

The 1990s were characterized by optimism regarding HIV/AIDS (see Figure 6.1). Scholars highlight the importance of positive thinking in American culture. In the case of life with disease, this refers to the belief that individual courage, a positive mindset, and willpower can help cope with or even overcome disease (Karpf, 1988; Lupton, 1999). This speaks to a mind-body connection (Ehrenreich, 2010; Lazarus, 1998) that is considered an important component of American culture to this day. According to Newman (2014), "encouragement of a cloying upbeat attitude is a phenomenon which extends right across American society. Historically, America has been pathologically life-affirming [...], but in the contemporary period positivity has become a central plank in American ideology" (p. 10). In Figure 6.1, the continuing influence of positive thinking is symbolized by the arrow starting in the mid- and late 1980s and going to the present day.

This development owes much to pharmaceutical companies, their products, and their advertising. With the increased availability of AZT, the first drug approved for treating HIV, the disease came to be perceived as chronic but manageable (Grover, 1992).

This shift in public perceptions was further bolstered through the advertising of drugs used in HIV therapy. In the 1990s, there was an upsurge in direct-to-consumer advertising for prescription drugs (DTCA) in general[3] (see Dan, 2015). Pharmaceutical companies manufacturing HIV drugs used extremely positive depictions of PLWHA in their advertising.[4] While this led to a written warning from the US Food and Drug Administration (FDA), the institution overseeing DTCA in the United States (see Jones, 1997), these ads were indisputably pushing the same agenda as activist efforts. Still, big pharma's approach must be seen in the context of potential economic gain: Given that the lifetime cost of treating an HIV infection was estimated at almost $380,000 in 2010 (CDC, 2013a), the HIV/AIDS market is very lucrative for pharmaceutical companies.

Another contributor to the shift in perceptions was the FDA decision to allow condom manufacturers to advertise that their products could help prevent sexually transmitted diseases (amfAR, 2011). HIV/AIDS now appeared preventable.

The media's interest in HIV/AIDS dropped accordingly (Swain, 2005; Treichler, 1999). Coverage became driven by routine events such as World AIDS Day (Bardhan, 2001, 2002). Occasional stories involving celebrities, scandals, and advances in treatment or in the quest for a cure also appeared (Pitts & Jackson, 1993; PSRA, 1996; Watts, 1993). On the positive side, the number of stories including a moral panic angle decreased considerably (Bardhan, 2001; Pickle, Quinn, & Brown, 2002). Also, coverage became less sensationalistic and more patient centered (Rogers et al., 1991). Horrid media images became less and less common (Treichler, 1999).

Since the 1990s, another major ideology in American culture began to be applied to HIV/AIDS—egalitarianism (see Corfe, 2008). As shown in Figure 6.1, egalitarianism was added to the mix; it did not necessarily replace earlier ideologies. Egalitarianism refers here to the idea that all people are made equal, and that they should have the same rights and opportunities. When egalitarianism is applied to HIV/AIDS, no distinction is made between "guilty" and "innocent" PLWHA; they are all equal. Also people are not deemed more or less worthy than others on the basis of their HIV status. This interpretation was promoted by countless activist efforts, most prominently by ACT UP (Gould, 2009). Also, following the FDA's warning to drug companies about their hyperbolic images in the 1990s, these companies began to present PLWHA in their advertising like everyday people (Scalvini, 2010).

Frames about People Living with HIV/AIDS: A Review

PLWHA have been portrayed in communication through four character frames[5] already identified in an earlier literature review: victim, survivor, carrier, and normal (see Dan & Coleman, 2014; Table 6.1). These four frames are dichotomized, in that categorizing someone as "normal" or "survivor" is defining them by contrast with their opposites, "carrier" and "victim," respectively (Goffman, 1963; Jones, 1997; Kitzinger, 1993; Ndiaye, 2014; Washington, 2006).

This typology most resembles that proposed by Lupton (1999), which included the AIDS victim, AIDS survivor, and AIDS carrier archetypes. One main difference was that she spoke of archetypes, where I prefer the term *character frames*.[6] Also, this typology includes a normal frame, a construct to which Lupton alluded—as the "antithesis" of the carrier frame (p. 38)—but did not further specify. Similarities also exist with other less well-known typologies (e.g., Albert, 1986; Hallet & Cannella, 1994; Pratt, Ha, & Pratt, 2002).

The Victim Frame

Based on the studies I review below, and expanding a definition we offered for its visual expression elsewhere (Dan & Coleman, 2014), I propose the following working definition of the victim frame (see Table 6.1):

> When people living with HIV/AIDS are presented through the victim frame, communicators choose words or visuals that emphasize the weakness in these people's bodies and personalities. The focus is placed on the negative aspects of their lives with disease, such as symptoms, treatment, side effects, and doctor's appointments on the one hand, and sadness, anxiety, shame, apathy, loneliness, and reduced self-determination on the other.

Several studies found constructs that align well with this definition, despite the use of different terminology. Most analyzed media samples, especially articles from general-interest media. In fact, only one study I could track found this frame in special-interest magazines. Specifically, Clarke, McLellan, and Hoffman-Goetz (2006) analyzed *Ebony* and *Essence*, which target readers of African descent in the United States and Canada. Scholars did not find this frame in public service announcements (PSAs).

Many studies discovered that media accounts of PLWHA emphasized their suffering. Here, physical and emotional pain appear to be interrelated. For instance, in her much-cited study, Lupton (1999) found that some of the press coverage of HIV/AIDS in Australia in the mid-1990s emphasized the deterioration of the health and emotional well-being of PLWHA (similar: Lupton, 1994a). At a time when the Australian government decided to legalize assisted suicide for terminally ill people, many articles told the story of individual people living with AIDS-related illnesses to exemplify the group of those potentially making use of this political recourse (Lupton, 1999). Similar findings were obtained in studies analyzing the media coverage of HIV/AIDS in other parts of the world, including the United States (Clarke et al., 2006; Sturken, 1997; Treichler, 1999), Great Britain (Kitzinger, 1995; Watney, 1990a, 1990b; Williams & Miller, 1995), India (D'Silva, Leichty, & Agarwal, 2011), and South Africa (Hodes, 2007). These studies suggest that many media accounts of HIV/AIDS described PLWHA as sick, frail, dependent on others, lonely, and full of negative emotions.

Most of the studies reviewed above were interested solely in the verbal aspects of communication about HIV and AIDS. Yet a relatively large number of early studies also paid attention to visuals, either exclusively (Crimp, 1992; Gilman, 1988; Watney, 1990b) or in addition to words (Hodes, 2007; Kitzinger, 1995; Lupton, 1999; Sturken, 1997; Treichler, 1999; Williams & Miller, 1995).

Many of these studies addressed the existence of images of PLWHA that suggested ill health. For instance, in her study of images of people living with AIDS in the United States, Grover (1992) encountered many pictures of suffering individuals with visible symptoms, such as images of "the bald and wasted AIDS patient with the feverish, haggard look, lying in his hospital bed (preferably with a few tubes up his nose)" (Drueilhe, 1988, p. 122; cited in Grover, 1992, p. 23). Similar tendencies were reported in other studies of the US media coverage (Albert, 1986; Treichler, 1999) and in studies from many other countries (Gilman, 1988), including the Philippines (Netter, 1992), Great Britain (Kitzinger, 1995; Watney, 1990a, 1990b; Wellings, 1988; Williams & Miller, 1995), South Africa (Hodes, 2007), and Germany (Wießner, 2004). Many scholars found that PLWHA were shown with medical equipment or in a medical setting. For example, Lupton (1994a) noted that PLWHA were depicted "lying passively in a hospital bed," "sitting listlessly in a wheelchair," or "connected to the machinery by various tubes and wires" (p. 44, 53). Similar results were obtained in South Africa (Hodes, 2007), the United States (Crimp, 1992), and Great Britain (Watney, 1990b). Crimp (1992), for instance, found that the "[m]ainstream coverage of AIDS [was] padded with portentous pictures of medical procedures—IV needles being inserted, doctors listening through stethoscopes, tinkering in laboratories" (p. 129).

Several authors referred to the many media visuals that implied a negative internal state by depicting PLWHA with negative expressions on their faces, isolated, and alone. For example, in various US media, the isolation of PLWHA was suggested by showing story protagonists backlit against windows, silhouetted against studio backdrops, or "at-the-window-watching-life-go-by-without-[them]" (Grover, 1992, p. 39).

Often they were shown alone (Cook & Colby, 1992; Crimp, 1992; Gilman, 1988; Juhasz, 1990; Lupton, 1999; Williams & Miller, 1995). In Great Britain, both Watney (1990b) and Kitzinger (1995) said that images abounded in the press of PLWHA who averted their gazes from the camera, who stared emptily or into the distance, or who looked "through" things. In Australia, Lupton (1999) described press photos showing PLWHA "looking pensive and morose" (p. 41) or "wiping away tears from [their] eyes" (p. 43; see also Lupton, 1994a). Visual tropes of isolation (Grover, 1992) appeared across countries, ranging from invisible, blurred or digitized faces, shots from behind or from above, to heavy backlighting or deep shadow (Cook & Colby, 1992; Crimp, 1992; Gilman, 1988; Grover, 1992; Kitzinger, 1991; Wellings, 1988).

Scholars differ in how they evaluated these techniques: Some acknowledged that they may have been meant to protect PLWHA from repercussions (Campbell, 2008; Grover, 1992; Kitzinger, 1991) while others deemed them dehumanizing and "othering" (Crimp, 1992; Gilman, 1988).

The Survivor Frame

Based on my review of literature, which I present below, and also drawing from our earlier definition proposed for its visual expression (Dan & Coleman, 2014), I propose the following working definition of the survivor frame (see Table 6.1):

> When people living with HIV/AIDS are presented through the survivor frame, communicators choose words or visuals that highlight the strength in these people's bodies and personalities. The focus is placed on the positive aspects of their lives. Generally, it is suggested that PLWHA are extremely healthy, active, and happy. Such accounts abound in mentions or portrayals of excellent physical fitness on the one hand, and a feeling of happiness, a sense of persistence and purpose in life, a desire to help others through volunteering or activism, a state of self-confidence, a fighting spirit, or a positive mindset on the other.

Many studies reported the description and portrayal of PLWHA in ways that correspond with the above definition. Again, just as it was for the victim frame, health status is linked to internal state.

The outlets in which this frame was identified in words or visuals include the general-interest media (Clarke et al., 2006; D'Silva et al., 2011; Hallet & Cannella, 1994; Lupton, 1994a, 1999; Sturken, 1997), special-interest and alternative publications (Clarke et al., 2006; Hallet & Cannella, 1994; Kitzinger, 1995), activist and nongovernmental organization (NGO) materials (Campbell, 2008; Crimp, 1992), and—especially—direct-to-consumer ads for HIV medication (Jones, 1997; Scalvini, 2010). Note that many of the studies reviewed in this section were also cited above, as these authors had not only identified the survivor frame in their samples but also its counterpart, the victim frame.

In her study of the Australian press coverage of HIV/AIDS, Lupton (1999) noticed that the availability of treatment for HIV allowed a new view of PLWHA to emerge in the media. Specifically, the media began to present PLWHA as strong-minded, vital, optimistic, proud, and courageous individuals who took good care of themselves. In Lupton's (1999) study, this frame appeared especially in connection to homosexual men and to the famous basketball player Magic Johnson. In a more recent Indian study, D'Silva and colleagues (2011) showed that the media coverage contained accounts of "heroes" and "heroines" (p. 75) who had "converted their HIV-positive status from a badge of social dishonor to a badge of honor that they accepted with pride" (p. 85). These stories presented PLWHA as commendable individuals who rejected the shame still associated with an HIV diagnosis, courageously fought the fight against their own disease, and got involved in activist work against stigma and discrimination (D'Silva et al., 2011).

Many scholars pointed to the existence of a visual expression of this frame, with PLWHA appearing healthy and full of energy, self-confident and presentable, or even beautiful or sensual (Campbell, 2008; Crimp, 1992; Jones, 1997; Kitzinger, 1995; Lupton, 1994a, 1999; Scalvini, 2010; Sturken, 1997). For example, in 1991, the British *Cosmopolitan* ran an article about Denise Hathaway, a woman living with HIV (Kitzinger, 1995). The article was entitled, "My name is Denise... I'm HIV-positive" and was illustrated with a glamour photo of the protagonist in which she looked healthy and attractive. Similarly, the Australian coverage contained various such photos, including that of a man "in an outdoor location, smiling broadly, looking healthy and fit, wearing sporting gear (shorts and a singlet) and carrying a bicycle over his shoulder" (Lupton, 1999, p. 44). Even more examples of a visual expression of the survivor frame in relation to PLWHA can be found in other contexts, to which I turn below.

Previous studies leave the impression that direct-to-consumer pharmaceutical ads (DTCA) long represented the "natural" location for the visual expression of the survivor frame. Indeed, Jones (1997) and Scalvini (2010) analyzed more than 50 print ads and found virtually no alternative visualizations. In Jones' (1997) words, PLWHA "appear[ed] as spectacles of health, possessing immaculate, athletic bodies," "healthy, handsome, smiling young men either in 'erotic' or 'semi-erotic' poses or in 'outdoorsy,' 'sporty' settings" (p. 397). These results were replicated in Scalvini's (2010) more recent study. Scalvini (2010) suggested that PLWHA—at least those taking the advertised medication—were depicted as self-confident individuals fighting and defeating the HI-virus, much like a rock climber conquering a mountain (the ad for Crixivan) or like a New York driver outsmarting others caught in a traffic jam (the ad for Atripla). Scalvini (2010) also drew attention to the way drug advertising had transformed the once "sick body" of PLWHA "into a body that was utopian, perfect, idealized, and even desirable" (p. 224).

Campbell (2008) reviewed the work of photographers such as Pep Bonet and Brent Stirton, who were entrusted with photographing PLWHA for use in NGO materials. Across these and other photographers' work, Campbell (2008) noticed a tendency to depict PLWHA in a way consistent with the survivor frame. PLWHA in treatment were depicted as vibrant, self-confident individuals. Some photographs only showed these individuals after the treatment had produced benefits. Others juxtaposed photos of PLWHA suffering with photos of them thriving (see Campbell, 2008).

Crimp (1992), in a side note to his analysis of Nixon's 1988 exhibition—which he criticized at length for the use of the victim frame—also offered some anecdotal evidence of the visual expression of the survivor frame in activist materials. Specifically, he recounted how on-site activists demonstrated against Nixon's way of depicting PLWHA by holding up alternative images. They showed photos of smiling or active PLWHA in their prime. One such photo showed a man speaking into microphones at a press conference. Its caption read, "My friend David Summers living with AIDS" (Crimp, 1992).

The Carrier Frame

I now turn to reviewing the literature where a carrier frame was identified. Also relying on our previous definition for its visual expression (Dan & Coleman, 2014) and the literature reviewed below, I define the carrier frame as follows (see Table 6.1):

> When people living with HIV/AIDS are presented through the carrier frame, communicators choose words or visuals that emphasize these people's perceived lack of self-control and dangerousness. The latter refers to the presentation of PLWHA as endangering others' health by maintaining the behavior that led to their infection—presented as volitional and deviant. They are presented as irresponsible, careless individuals who have brought disease upon themselves and who now spread disease either due to negligence or intentionally.

An impressive number of studies identified constructs consistent with this definition, which I review below in more detail. As a general remark, this frame was found exclusively in analyses of general-interest media and in PSAs; I found no evidence of this frame SIPs.

Many early studies analyzing the general-interest media coverage at the beginning of the epidemic found that PLWHA were presented in the media and in PSAs as individuals who got the virus because they lacked self-control over their cravings for sex and drugs. Consequently, PLWHA were constructed as having no one to blame for their plight but themselves (e.g., Hallet & Cannella, 1994; Hammond, 1997).

First, pertaining to the idea that PLWHA are unable to control their drives, a wide range of studies reported how general-interest media accounts established causal links between HIV/AIDS and promiscuity or drug use. In both words and visuals, the suffering upon contagion was presented as divine punishment for the perceived violation of social, moral, and religious standards (Kitzinger, 1995). Several authors explained how photos of attractive young men "indulging" *[sic]* in gay discos or bathhouses were juxtaposed with photos of them suffering in hospital beds (see Clarke, 1992; Crimp, 1992; D'Silva et al., 2011; de Souza, 2007; Kitzinger, 1995; Wellings, 1988). Such stigmatizing coverage of gay PLWHA seems to have decreased over time, yet this frame was reported in later studies with reference to promiscuity (regardless of sexual orientation) and drug use (see also Dan & Coleman, 2014; Lupton, 1999). For example, Treichler (1999) noticed that general-interest US stories about HIV/AIDS were routinely illustrated with a photo of a "Third World prostitute, in red" (p. 133). In PSAs, too, PLWHA were often described and depicted as immoral, tempting individuals wanting to spread the virus (see Gausset, Mogensen, Yameogo, Berthé, & Konaté, 2012; Gilman, 1995).

Second, consistent with the idea that PLWHA endanger others' health due to negligence or out of vengefulness, many studies suggested that the general-interest media and PSAs presented PLWHA as disease spreaders. Many analyzed the US general-interest coverage (Albert, 1986; Juhasz, 1993; Sacks, 1996; Sontag, 1989; Sturken, 1997; Treichler, 1988b, 1999; Williams & Miller, 1995), but this frame also occurred elsewhere, including in Papua New Guinea (Cullen & Callaghan, 2010), Britain (Kitzinger, 1993; Wellings, 1988), and other Western countries (Lupton, 1994b). Lupton (1999) provided a rich list of examples. She explained how Australian media sometimes singled out for coverage drug users with HIV who did not properly discard their syringes; an obstetrician living with HIV who did not disclose his status to the women on whom he performed surgery; and various PLWHA who stabbed others with their syringes, who bit other people, or who seduced and contaminated unknowing sexual partners (Lupton, 1999). On top of this, critical scholars pointed out that it was often women living with HIV/AIDS who were presented in the media coverage (Kitzinger, 1993) and in PSAs (Gilman, 1995) as disease spreaders for contaminating their unborn children (Sacks, 1996) or—in the case of commercial sex workers—their unsuspecting sexual partners (Sacks, 1996; Watney, 1990a). The idea that PLWHA are contagious was sometimes conveyed visually through the use of protective gear by those establishing physical contact with them (Albert, 1986).

The Normal Frame

Finally, I turn to the studies that found descriptions and depictions of PLWHA consistent with the normal frame. Based on these studies, and on our earlier definition (Dan & Coleman, 2014), I propose that the normal frame presents PLWHA as follows (see Table 6.1):

> When people living with HIV/AIDS are presented through the normal frame, words or visuals underscore that they are not to blame for contracting the virus, present the ways in which PLWHA go on with their lives despite disease, have a support system, and feel generally healthy and happy. This presentation is not hyperbolic; rather, it acknowledges that PLWHA may experience bad days both in terms of physical and emotional well-being, but that these are outnumbered by the good ones. Correspondingly, photos resemble those in family albums and show individuals who seem generally healthy and wear a neutral to positive facial expression, and/or are surrounded by friends, loved ones, or pets.

This is a relatively new frame to be applied to PLWHA. At the beginning of the epidemic, this frame was mostly encountered in SIPs in the United States (Grover, 1992). Later on, as it became clear that women, children, and heterosexual men could also contract HIV/AIDS, the general-interest US news started to convey this frame, too (Cook & Colby, 1992; Juhasz, 1990). It was also reported in the general-interest media coverage of other countries, including South Africa (Hodes, 2007). The normal frame was also encountered in NGO materials (Campbell, 2008; Olesen, 2012). Finally, according to a recent study, this frame was featured in the visuals of DTCA for the antiretroviral drugs used in HIV therapy (Scalvini, 2010), suggesting that pharmaceutical companies made efforts to implement the FDA's requests to tone down their visuals (for comparison, see "The Survivor Frame" above).

A first component of this frame is the notion that these PLWHA contracted HIV/AIDS through no fault of their own. For instance, they might be described as having been deceived by partners whom they trusted or as not having had any possibility to protect themselves from contagion (i.e., mother-to-child transmission). It is mostly women, hemophiliacs, and infants/children who were freed of blame in the media (Crimp, 1992; de Souza, 2007; Hoffman-Goetz, Friedman, & Clarke, 2005; Lupton, 1994a; Montgomery, 1990; Wellings, 1988), PSAs (Gilman, 1995), and in NGO materials (Olesen, 2012). The women selected for coverage through this lens were typically white, married, middle class, and heterosexual (Lupton, 1999). Yet, two studies suggested that homosexual men can also receive this type of media treatment (Crimp, 1992; Lupton, 1999). Being constructed as free of blame, these PLWHA also seem noncontagious, as denoted by the fact that no protective gear was used by those interacting with them (Albert, 1986).

A second component of this frame is the idea that PLWHA go on with their lives despite disease. Presenting PLWHA in this way meets activist demands to see the "person first," not the medical condition the person lives with (Quinlan, 2014). PLWHA were described as whole people. Specifically, instead of being reduced to their disease, their identities were defined by other aspects of their lives, such as work, hobbies, family, or love life (Campbell, 2008; Grover, 1992).

A third element of this frame is the average nature and appearance of PLWHA. For instance, Scalvini (2010) found that several drug companies used images of PLWHA engaging in simple daily activities (e.g., doing laundry); looking as they did 5 years after the diagnosis; and reaching life milestones, such as getting married. As one service organization director said in a TV interview, "We know the individuals, and they look a lot like you, they look a lot like me" (cited in Crimp, 1992, p. 122). Several camera techniques were considered to strengthen this impression through their use of eye-level shots and medium camera angles (Juhasz, 1990).

A fourth and final element of this frame is the average internal state. The PLWHA seemed to cope just fine with their diagnosis. They seemed involved in their health care (Treichler, 1999), as though managing HIV only played a minimal role in their lives (Scalvini, 2010). Also, it was verbally and visually suggested that they have a solid support system. For instance, several studies reported having found visuals of PLWHA engaging in (physical) contact with people or animals (Cook & Colby, 1992; Crimp, 1992; Gilman, 1988; Grover, 1992; Treichler, 1999). Similarly, NGO photographers preferred showing PLWHA with loved ones in a domestic setting (Campbell, 2008; Kilian, 2014; McCullin, 2004).

A summary of the literature reviewed in this subchapter is offered in Table 6.1. It appears there is a clear verbal and visual expression of each of the four frames, along the lines of physical health and fitness, internal state, contagion scenario, and social status.

Table 6.1 Key Components of the Four Frames According to Previous Studies

	Victim		*Survivor*		*Carrier*		*Normal*	
	Verbal components	*Visual components*	*Verbal components*	*Visual components*	*Verbal components*	*Visual components*	*Verbal components*	*Visual components*
Health and fitness	Poor (symptoms, treatment, side-effects, doctor's visits)	Poor (symptoms, signs of disease, medical equipment, pills)	Excellent (very healthy, sporty, health conscious)	Excellent (no signs of disease, presentable/ beautiful, workout)			Average (good days and bad days)	Average (neither bursting with health nor sick)
Internal state	Negative (reduced self-determination, loneliness, negative emotions)	Negative (looking away, passive, alone, negative facial expression)	Excellent (fighting spirit, activism, very happy and self-confident)	Excellent (smiling, confident-looking, very positive facial expression)			Average (cope well with diagnosis)	Average (neutral till positive facial expression)
Contagion scenario					"Guilty" (no self-control, volitional, deviant behavior, self-inflicted)	"Guilty" (deviant behavior depicted)	"Innocent" (free of blame)	—
Social status					Outcast (deviant, disease spreader)	Visual tropes of isolation; no contact to others or contact with protective gear	Acceptable (like everybody else; support system)	Shown with approving others; does everyday activities

Research Questions, Hypotheses, and Strategy of Analysis

This study addressed 10 hypotheses and two research questions. Further below, they are offered along with a short recap of the theoretical considerations that led to the proposal of each (for an overview, see Table 6.2).

The hypotheses and research questions in this study were addressed using Chi-square/Fisher's Exact and *F* tests. The procedures were crosstabs and analyses of variance (ANOVA).

For crosstabs larger than 2 x 2, a column proportions test—a *z*-test—using the Bonferroni correction was conducted to adjust the *p*-values in such a way to correct for multiple comparisons. Afterward, column proportions were compared pairwise; subscript letters indicated pairs that were significantly different. Cramér's V was used as an indicator of effect size (Cohen, 1988, p. 222). The interpretation of the Cramér's V as denoting an effect size that is small, medium, or large depends on the degrees of freedom (df). For instance, Cramér's V = .30 denotes a medium effect with one degree of freedom but a large effect with three or more degrees of freedom. Whenever 20% or more of the cells had fewer than five observations each, the corrected *p*-value as returned by the Fisher's Exact Test was reported instead of that provided by the Chi-square test of significance (Cochran, 1954). Furthermore, whenever SPSS was unable to calculate the exact values due to computational limits—this happens when the overall sample size is large but some expected counts are small—the Monte Carlo Test was used instead of Fisher's. This option uses approximations to the exact *p*-values. I increased the confidence intervals for the Monte Carlo *p*-values to 99.99% and the number of samples to 1,000,000. This allowed me to obtain the exact *p*-values to a given number of decimals. According to SPSS, one can be "fairly confident that this value is the exact significance." (IBM Support, 2016).

The ANOVAs were one-way, two-way, or three-way, depending on the number of independent variables included in the tests. When ANOVAs were used, the analysis strategy involved a test of homogeneity of variance and post hoc tests. When the Levene test suggested that the assumption of homogeneity of variance was tenable, the *F* value returned by the ANOVA was reported, and post-hoc paired comparisons were computed using the Tukey HSD post-hoc test. However, when the Levene statistic suggested the assumption of equal variance had been violated, Welch's robust tests for equality of means were used and post-hoc paired comparisons were calculated using the Dunnett C test, which does not assume equal variance. Eta squared (η^2) was reported as an estimate of effect size whenever significant differences occurred. The effect sizes are typically interpreted as follows: small = .01, medium = .06, and large = .14 (Cohen, 1988, p. 222).

The literature reviewed at the beginning of this chapter suggested that at some point, all four frames of interest here were conveyed in news, both

Table 6.2 Overview of Research Questions and Hypotheses in This Study

Level of Analysis	*Object of Investigation*	*Research Question/Hypothesis*
Verbal frames/ visual frames	Differences in framing based on the communication context (news, SIPs, PSAs)	H1a: The victim and the carrier frames will be used significantly more in news than in SIPs and PSAs. H1b: The normal and the survivor frames will be conveyed significantly more in SIPs and PSAs than in news.
	Frame building (differences in framing based on news sources/photo sources)	H2a: The verbal frames conveyed in news will differ significantly among the news sources used. H2b: The visual frames conveyed in news will differ significantly among the photo sources used.
	Differences in framing based on the characteristics of the target audience and/or the goal of communication	H3a: The normal, survivor, and victim frames will be used significantly more in news from states characterized by low conservatism, low religiosity, high HIV/AIDS prevalence, and high urbanism than in their counterparts. H3b: The carrier frame will be used significantly more in news from states characterized by high conservatism, high religiosity, low HIV/AIDS prevalence, and low urbanism than in their counterparts. H4: The normal and the survivor frames will be used significantly more in SIPs targeted at PLWHA than in those directed at African Americans and the LGBT community. RQ1: Do the frames conveyed in PSAs differ significantly based on the type of PSA (prevention, treatment, anti-stigma)?
	Differences in framing based on the characteristics of the PLWHA (gender, race/ ethnicity, and sexuality)	H5a: The victim and the carrier frames will be used significantly more for PLWHA who are female, homosexual/bisexual, or non-white than for those who are male, heterosexual, or white, respectively. H5b: The normal and the survivor frames will be used significantly more for PLWHA who are male, heterosexual, or white than for those who are female, homosexual/bisexual, or non-white, respectively.
Visual frames	Differences in framing based on the nonverbal behavior of the PLWHA	H6: The nonverbal behavior exhibited by PLWHA depicted through the survivor and normal frames will be significantly more positive than that displayed by PLWHA framed as victim or carrier.
	Differences in framing based on structural features (camera angle, camera distance)	H7a: Normal, victim, and carrier frames will use significantly more eye-level camera angles than survivor frames. H7b: Survivor frames will use significantly more low-level camera angles than normal, victim, and carrier frames. H7c: Victim frames will use significantly more high-level camera angles than normal, victim, and carrier frames. H8a: Normal and survivor frames will use significantly more medium and long shots than victim and carrier frames. H8b: Victim and carrier frames will use significantly more close-ups than normal and survivor frames.

(*Continued*)

Level of Analysis	*Object of Investigation*	*Research Question/Hypothesis*
The interplay between verbal frames and visual frames	Differences in the frame congruence ratio based on…	
	… the communication context (news, SIPs, PSAs)	H9: The verbal-visual frame congruence ratio will be significantly higher in PSAs than in SIPs and news.
	… the characteristics of the target audience and/or the goal of communication	RQ2: Does the verbal-visual frame congruence ratio differ significantly based on the characteristics of the state publishing the newspaper, the target audience of SIPs, or the PSA type?
	… the verbal frame	H10: The verbal-visual congruence ratio will vary significantly according to the verbal frame conveyed.

through words and through visuals (e.g., Crimp, 1992; Treichler, 1999), although the intensity to which they were transmitted varied greatly over time. PSAs and SIPs were much more focused and used only a limited number of frames (e.g., Gilman, 1995; Grover, 1992). Moreover, the research reviewed in Chapter 4 suggested that advocates generally transmitted frames intended to help them achieve certain goals (e.g., Carragee & Roefs, 2004; Hänggli & Kriesi, 2012; Pan & Kosicki, 2001). The advocacy materials analyzed in this study—special-interest publications (SIPs) directed at subpopulations most affected by the epidemic and PSAs aiming to contain the epidemic partly by normalizing HIV/AIDS—are likely to have an interest in portraying PLWHA in a positive light. On the other hand, journalists are more likely to try to be objective and paint a complex picture by addressing both the good and the bad. From this perspective, the following hypotheses seemed plausible. Because the frames are categorical measures, these hypotheses were tested using a Chi-square test of significance with a Bonferroni correction:

H1a: The victim and the carrier frames will be used significantly more in news than in SIPs and PSAs.

H1b: The normal and the survivor frames will be conveyed significantly more in SIPs and PSAs than in news.

The answer to the above hypotheses should reveal which verbal and visual frames were preferred by journalists and advocates. These insights were used next to investigate the connection between frames in news and the use of certain news sources, following the lead of Strömbäck et al. (2013) and Dimitrova and Strömbäck (2012) (see Chapter 4). In an attempt to expand the focus, I investigated not just whether verbal news frames differed among the news sources used—as these authors did—but also whether the visual frames differed among the photo sources used (i.e., news sources providing visuals). A Chi-square test of significance and a Fisher's Exact Test with a Bonferroni correction were used to examine the following hypotheses:

H2a: The verbal frames conveyed in news will differ significantly among the news sources used.

H2b: The visual frames conveyed in news will differ significantly among the photo sources used.

Next, the focus was directed at the extent to which statistically significant differences existed between the occurrence of frames—verbal and visual—and the characteristics of the population in the states in which the newspapers in the sample were issued (i.e., the community structure). Previous research suggested that PLWHA may be treated more harshly by those who are more conservative (Doka, 1997), more religious

(Muturi & An, 2010), who live in rural areas (Dhooper & Royse, 1989; Mondragón, Kirkman-Life, & Schneller, 1991), and/or in areas with low HIV/AIDS prevalence (Bates, 2007; Clawson, Strine, & Waltenburg, 2003; Krishnan, Durrah, & Winkler, 1997; Patterson, 2014; Rim, Lee, & Han, 2009; Temoshok, Grade, & Zich, 1988). Despite contradictory research findings on the influence of individual differences on journalists' reporting (see for a recent review, Shoemaker & Reese, 2014), the community structure approach (Pollock, 2007) allows the assumption that newspapers targeted at audiences sharing these characteristics may frame PLWHA differently than newspapers targeted at audiences with the opposite characteristics. In other words, it is possible that local news people acknowledged how their communities were made up and that this prevented journalists across the United States from covering HIV/AIDS in a homogeneous way. For instance, Liebler and Bendix (1996) found that the framing of an environmental controversy (cutting vs. saving old-growth forests) was consistently pro-cut in news from areas were many people worked in the timber industry, and explained that "[r]eporters may also have been responding to the social environment in which they were working" (p. 59). Other studies identified the racial/ethnic structure of communities as one common potential influencer, but potential confounding variables were not always taken into account (see for a review McLemore, 2015). A Chi-square test of significance and Fisher's Exact Test with a Bonferroni correction were used to investigate the following:

H3a: The normal, survivor, and victim frames will be used significantly more in news from states characterized by low conservatism, low religiosity, high HIV/AIDS prevalence, and high urbanism than in their counterparts.

H3b: The carrier frame will be used significantly more in news from states characterized by high conservatism, high religiosity, low HIV/AIDS prevalence, and low urbanism than in their counterparts.

The next hypothesis predicted differences in framing based on the target audiences of special-interest publications. The SIPs in the sample were directed at PLWHA, at African Americans, and at members of the LGBT community, respectively. The first group of readers was most directly affected by HIV/AIDS, whereas only some of the readers of the other types of SIPs may have lived with HIV/AIDS. Against this background, I tested the following hypothesis using a Fisher's Exact Test with a Bonferroni correction:

H4: The normal and the survivor frames will be used significantly more in SIPs targeted at PLWHA than in those directed at African Americans and the LGBT community.

The sample for this study included not just "classical" PSAs (i.e., those aiming to contain the HIV epidemic by preventing its further spread, but also PSAs promoting treatment and advocating against stigma and the discrimination of PLWHA. Given the different goals of these PSAs, it was conceivable that prevention PSAs would convey different frames than treatment and anti-stigma PSAs. The literature reviewed above suggested that, in the early days, public health communicators did not shy away from transmitting carrier frames—in other words, from suggesting that PLWHA were out-of-control disease spreaders (Gausset et al., 2012; Gilman, 1995). However, predicting that prevention PSAs would convey carrier frames would mean assuming that decades of research showing the detrimental effects of stigma and discrimination on containing the epidemic (e.g., Aggleton & Parker, 2002; Alonzo & Reynolds, 1995) went unnoticed by public health communicators. It was difficult to predict exactly how the frames in prevention PSAs would differ from those in treatment and anti-stigma PSAs. Thus, I asked the following research question, which was addressed using Fisher's Exact Test with a Bonferroni correction:

RQ1: Do the frames conveyed in PSAs differ significantly based on the type of PSA (prevention, treatment, anti-stigma)?

Previous research suggested there may be a double bind in the way PLWHA are treated in communication and in real life. Specifically, there was a chance that women, homosexual/bisexual individuals, and racial/ethnic minorities were described and portrayed in more negative ways than their counterparts. Most studies suggested this was the case, though exceptions existed (Coleman & Hatley Major, 2014; Dan & Coleman, 2014). As described above in depth, the carrier frame was more often conveyed for women living with HIV/AIDS than for their (heterosexual) male counterparts, both in the media coverage and in PSAs (Gilman, 1995; Kitzinger, 1993; Sacks, 1996; Watney, 1990a). On the other hand, homosexual men were often presented through the carrier frame, especially in the media coverage (Clarke, 1992; Crimp, 1992; D'Silva et al., 2011; de Souza, 2007; Kitzinger, 1995; Wellings, 1988). Also, most research to date found that PLWHA belonging to racial and ethnic minorities were often presented in more negative ways than white PLWHA in the media (Treichler, 1999) and in PSAs (DeJong, Wolf, & Austin, 2001). Such detrimental treatment of women, homosexual/bisexual individuals, and racial/minorities may be most readily apparent in the way these groups are framed visually. The literature reviewed in Chapter 2 suggested that nowadays, presenting a certain subpopulation in a discriminatory way is more likely to occur visually than verbally (see Burgoon, Buller, & Woodall, 1996; Coleman, 2010;

Messaris & Abraham, 2001). With this in mind, I used a Fisher's Exact Test (Monte Carlo method) with a Bonferroni correction to check the following:

H5a: The victim and the carrier frames will be used significantly more for PLWHA who are female, homosexual/bisexual, or non-white than for those who are male, heterosexual, or white, respectively.
H5b: The normal and the survivor frames will be used significantly more for PLWHA who are male, heterosexual, or white than for those who are female, homosexual/bisexual, or non-white, respectively.

As explained below in more depth, three types of information were extracted from the visuals for this study: photo content, nonverbal behavior, and structural features (i.e., camera distance and camera-angle settings). At the time when this study was conducted, researchers were rather divided in their assessment of which of these characteristics qualified as frame components and which did not. More precisely, the status of nonverbal behavior and structural features was contested. As reviewed in Chapter 3, researchers in the symbolic-semiotic tradition argued that these visual characteristics were relevant to framing (see Grabe, 1996; Moriarty & Popovich, 1991; Rodriguez & Dimitrova, 2011). Other scholars cautioned against considering every conceivable variation in a visual as a frame component. Grittmann (2013) argued that such a tendency would only weaken the explanatory power of visual framing. To account for this difference of opinion, variables from all three categories—photo content, nonverbal behavior, and structural features—were submitted to a reliability analysis (Cronbach's alpha) designed to help identify visual frames. (Details on the index building are offered in Results.) In case the reliability analysis revealed that these variables did not occur together as expected—i.e., that they did not qualify as frame components—I proposed a hypothesis designed to test whether or not significant differences between the frames and the valence of nonverbal behavior existed. This circumstance materialized. With the survivor and normal frames being more positive than the victim and carrier frames, an *F*-test and Tukey HSD post-hoc tests were used to test the following:

H6: The nonverbal behavior exhibited by PLWHA depicted through the survivor and normal frames will be significantly more positive than that displayed by PLWHA framed as victim or carrier.

As explained in Chapter 3, different camera angles have different connotations (Banning & Coleman, 2009; Bell & Milic, 2002; Berger, 1981; Coleman, 2010; Grabe & Bucy, 2009; Jewitt & Oyama, 2012; Messaris, 1997). Specifically, when people are depicted using a low shot (i.e., the viewer is looking up at the person depicted), they are likely to seem more powerful than when high shots are used (i.e., the viewer is looking down at the protagonist); eye-level shots are considered neutral (see Table 3.1). Previous research suggested that photographers and camera people may vary camera angles to suggest that politicians are powerful or weak (see Grabe & Bucy, 2009). However, these professionals may be less vested in conveying such latent meanings when it comes to PLWHA, or they may reject high angles as too contemptuous or low angles as hyperbolic. With survivor being the most positive frame accounted for in this study, I resorted to a Fisher's Exact Test with a Bonferroni correction to test the following:

H7a: Normal, victim, and carrier frames will use significantly more eye-level camera angles than survivor frames.
H7b: Survivor frames will use significantly more low-level camera angles than normal, victim, and carrier frames.
H7c: Victim frames will use significantly more high-level camera angles than normal, victim, and carrier frames.

Moreover, the four visual frames investigated in this study could have used different camera distances. Most research into camera distances was conducted in the field of political communication. In Chapter 3, I explained how variations in camera distance make the subject seem closer to or farther away from the viewer, both spatially and socially (see Coleman, 2010; Grabe & Bucy, 2009). As summarized in Table 3.1, for politicians, scholars typically considered a medium shot neutral, a long shot negative, and close-ups positive. The connotations of close-ups may differ for politicians and PLWHA, however. The person depicted through close-ups "enters" the personal space of the viewer. This can produce closeness and familiarity (as is typically assumed in political communication studies) or, quite the contrary, hostility. This is something Fiske (2011) addressed at length. In his view, close-ups—extreme close-ups, in particular—can be alienating. He argued that extreme close-ups are "a codified way for representing villainy" (Fiske, 2011, p. 6). In his own study of televised images, Fiske found that extreme close-ups were "more likely to be used to portray villains than heroes" (Fiske, 2011, p. 33).

From this perspective, it seemed unlikely that communicators would choose close-ups to convey the frames that present PLWHA in a good light (i.e., normal or survivor). Rather, it appeared more probable that close-ups would be used to depict PLWHA going through a rough patch—by zooming in on teary faces (see Kitch, 2009), for example. Similarly, close-ups could be used to portray PLWHA accused or convicted of crimes, as studies found that police-produced mug shots reproduced in the media often used close-ups (Trautman, 2004). Conversely, it was possible that the negative frames for PLWHA would not use long shots. By showing the surroundings of the PLWHA—their homes, for instance—long shots may actually be used to convey normal and survivor frames—that is, when communicators try to present PLWHA as average or as extraordinary people. For these reasons, I posed the following hypotheses that were tested using a Fisher's Exact Test with a Bonferroni correction:

H8a: Normal and survivor frames will use significantly more medium and long shots than victim and carrier frames.
H8b: Victim and carrier frames will use significantly more close-ups than normal and survivor frames.

Previous research has highlighted mass communication in which communication through the verbal channel was neutral or even sympathetic toward PLWHA, while the accompanying visuals were discriminatory and accusing (Cook, 1989; Hodes, 2007; Treichler, 1999). The last hypotheses and research questions addressed in this study referred more specifically to the relationship between verbal and visual frames. To investigate the extent to which verbal and visual frames in one message conveyed similar meanings—something I called the verbal-visual frame congruence ratio—the formula proposed in Chapter 5 was used. Applying this formula to the data resulted in a new interval-level variable that was used in subsequent analyses (see Chapter 5, Step 6).

The first hypothesis using this newly computed variable started from the observation that, generally, PSAs are decidedly and openly persuasive (Faden & Faden, 1978), whereas news and SIPs are not. Pairing the insights from Chapters 2 and 4, it seemed plausible to assume that public health communicators would put more effort into transmitting verbal frames that were reinforced by the accompanying visual frames, and vice versa. I used a Welch's F-test and Dunnett's C post-hoc tests to address the following hypothesis:

H9: The verbal-visual frame congruence ratio will be significantly higher in PSAs than in SIPs and news.

Next, I investigated whether the verbal-visual frame congruence ratio differed according to the characteristics of the medium under scrutiny (the same characteristics used for H2 and H3, see above). As this type of research had never been done before, no solid prediction could be made. I posed the following research question, which was addressed using F-tests:

RQ2: Does the verbal-visual frame congruence ratio differ significantly based on the characteristics of the state publishing the newspaper, the target audience of SIPs, or the PSA type?

The last hypothesis tested whether the congruence ratio depended on the frame conveyed. Again, this was new territory, and specific predictions were impossible. It seemed plausible, however, that communicators would pay more attention to verbal-visual frame congruence for some frames than others. This is because they might be more able or more eager to transmit some frames than others. I thus posed the following hypothesis, which I tested using an *F*-test and Tukey HSD post-hoc tests:

H10: The verbal-visual congruence ratio will vary significantly according to the verbal frame conveyed.

Methodology

Sample

As shown in Table 6.3, the verbal framing of 656 people living with HIV/AIDS (PLWHA) was analyzed in news, special-interest/niche publications (SIPs), and public service announcements (PSAs). In these same contexts, the visual framing of 580 PLWHA was investigated. The numbers were not identical, because some materials in the sample did not contain both verbal and visual frames.

The goal was to select a highly diverse sample of articles published on the websites of local, metropolitan, and international newspapers; of news magazines; of SIPs, and PSAs. First, this allows the testing of the proposed approach to integrative framing analyses on the communication contexts that are most commonly investigated in our discipline. Second, a diverse sample helps identify the contexts in which integrative framing analyses are most relevant (due to differences between verbal frames and visual frames). Local newspapers were included given the tremendous attention[7] to health-related matters in local media (Fitzgerald, 1997; Schwitzer, 1992; Tanner, 2004) and local news' popularity among Americans (Coulson, Lacy, & Wilson, 2000; Mitchell, 2014). Finally, including messages conveying both news frames and advocacy frames in the analysis allows the investigation of frame building—something very much neglected in current literature (see Chapter 4).

Table 6.3 Sample Overview

	News Articles (n = 126)	*SIPs Articles (n = 67)*	*PSAs (n = 94)*	*Total*
PLHWA in the verbal component	242	311	103	656
PLHWA in the visual component	204	230	146	580

News articles were selected from the top three online newspapers in each of the nine geographic divisions of the United States[8] (by digital circulation) and the top websites of news magazines (*TIME* and *Newsweek*). These 29 websites were searched for news stories containing the term "HIV" between June 1, 2013, and June 1, 2014. The articles returned by the search were included in the sample only if they contained at least one photo showing an individual identified in the surrounding text, especially in the photo caption, as living with HIV/AIDS. Almost all these news websites featured articles meeting this criterion. The exceptions were the websites of *Union Leader* (New Hampshire), *Burlington Free Press* (Vermont), *Argus Leader* (South Dakota), and *Newsweek*. Only articles from the remaining 24 news sites were included in the sample, namely, *The Arizona Republic* (Arizona), *Missoulian* (Montana), *The Salt-Lake Tribune* (Utah), *Los Angeles Times* (California), *The Oregonian* (Oregon), *Chicago Sun-Times* (Illinois), *Plain Dealer* (Ohio), *Milwaukee Journal Sentinel* (Wisconsin), *Star Tribune* (Minnesota), *St. Louis Post-Dispatch* (Missouri), *The Wichita Eagle* (Kansas), *New York Post* (New York), *The New York Times* (New York), *Newark Star-Ledger* (New Jersey), *Washington Post* (District of Columbia), *Charlotte Observer* (North Carolina), *Tampa Bay Times* (Florida), *Montgomery Advertiser* (Alabama), *The Courier-Journal* (Kentucky), *The Tennessean* (Tennessee), *Arkansas Democrat Gazette* (Arkansas), *Dallas Morning News* (Texas), *Wall Street Journal* (international), and *TIME* magazine. These news websites are run from states different in terms of political views, religiousness, HIV/AIDS rates, and rural/urban ratio (see Appendix).

For the articles in SIPs, the websites of magazines directed at subpopulations most affected by HIV/AIDS—namely, African Americans, Hispanics/Latinos, and gay and bisexual men—were searched for articles containing the word "HIV" (or "VIH" on the Spanish websites) and illustrated with at least one photo of a genuine PLWHA between June 1, 2013, and June 1, 2014. Specifically, these were the websites of *Ebony, Essence, People en Español, Latina, Advocate*, and *OUT* magazines. No articles on the websites of *People en Español* and *Latina* met the criterion for selection; all the other publications were kept. Additionally, the *POZ* magazine was included in the sample. *POZ* is a glossy magazine for people living with HIV/AIDS. As many more articles on the *POZ* website were illustrated with photos of genuine PLWHA than could be included in the present analysis, the print editions of the magazine were used instead; they were available online on ISSUU.com.

To collect PSAs for analysis, the websites of the Centers for Disease Control and Prevention (CDC) and of Greater than AIDS were searched. Again, the criterion for selection was that the PSA showed a PLWHA who was also referenced in the text. Accordingly, PSAs from five campaigns were selected, two from the CDC and three from Greater than AIDS. They were *Let's Stop HIV Together, HIV Treatment Works, I Got Tested*, *Deciding Moments*, and *Empowered*.

Data Collection

Prior to the development of the codebooks, the verbal component of the materials in my sample had to be disjoined from its visual counterpart.[9] (This corresponds to Step 1 in Figure 5.1.) Each article and PSA in the sample was split into its words and its visuals. All photos showing at least one PLWHA as identified in the text were included in the visual framing analysis. For news articles and articles in SIPs, a student archived all information available in the photo captions before the splitting began. The photo captions were included in the verbal analysis. The part of the photo caption including photo credits was also archived separately, together with the corresponding ID number of the photo, for later use in the coding of photo sourcing. When no credits were provided in the photo caption, the student was instructed to look for this information on the side of the photo or underneath the title of the article. Cues such as "courtesy of," "photographs by," "portraits by," and so forth were used to identify credits. For print PSAs, the student typed all words on the posters. To relate the verbal frames to the visual frames in the analysis (Step 6), the verbal component and the visual component were assigned matching identification numbers (see Figure 5.1).

The selection of approaches to the identification of verbal frames and visual frames, respectively, was another prerequisite for developing the two codebooks. (This satisfies Step 2 shown in Figure 5.1.)

To identify verbal frames, two of the available approaches were connected. First, the deductive approach was chosen because the four frames (victim, survivor, carrier, normal) seemed likely to have been described in previous studies. The literature reviewed at the beginning of this chapter clearly suggested that this assumption was correct. Yet, unlike most studies using this approach, the present one does not use holistic measures in order to reduce the risk of overlooking frames that were not anticipated.[10] Thus, this study combined the deductive approach with the manual-clustering approach (see Chapter 3). The latter allowed the separation of the frames of interest into elements to be coded separately rather than holistically. Unlike Matthes and Kohring (2008), no attempts were made to align each frame component to the four framing functions[11] proposed by Entman (1993). This endeavor may be suitable for the framing of issues, but it is not suitable for the framing of people. Instead, explaining how the frames of interest structure social reality seemed more meaningful. In sum, combining these two approaches evaded the inflexibility of the deductive approach and capped the open nature of the manual-clustering approach.

To identify visual frames, the symbolic-semiotic approach[12] was combined with the denotative deductive approach. This combination was not so much intended to compensate for the flaws of the respective approaches but rather to account both for photo content and for latent meaning conveyed by photo characteristics beyond content (see Table 3.2). These two approaches seemed suitable, given that this study set out to identify generic frames using quantitative methods. My interest in generic frames is justified by my understanding of frames as recurring patterns of interpretation that are largely independent of the topic analyzed. I justify my preference for quantitative methods with the need to cope with a relatively large sample with limited resources. However, this study drew in part on inductive methods and also tried to reveal latent meaning (details are offered below); the former is more typical for qualitative studies, the latter for critical methods.

Codebook Development

In keeping with Step 3 in Figure 5.1, two interconnected codebooks were developed: one for the words, one for the visuals.

In addition to variables immediately relevant to the research questions and hypotheses, the codebooks contained variables recording identifying information for the coded material (ID number, title, source, link, and date) and for the person living with HIV/AIDS to which the coding referred (ID number, name, gender, sexuality, age, and race).

The variables concerning the research questions and hypotheses can be divided into two major groups. Variables meant to record information potentially relevant to the framing of PLWHA belonged to the first group; the second group consisted of variables informing about news sourcing and photos sourcing.

The framing variables (i.e., those belonging to the first group) were used for all communication contexts under scrutiny—news, SIPs, and PSAs. They represented the main part of each codebook. The sourcing variables were only employed for news stories in the sample, as they relate to news frame building.

For the framing variables, the unit of analysis was the individual PLWHA referred to in the text or shown in the photo. For the sourcing variables, the unit of analysis was the verbal component of every article or the individual photograph. Coders were instructed to go through the codebook once for each PLWHA appearing in the verbal or visual component of each article and print PSA. This means that at least one—but possibly more—PLWHA was coded for each article and PSA. This was an attempt to make room for the possibility that more frames would appear in a text and in a photo (see Dahmen, 2009; Matthes, 2007), given that framing is considered socially relevant only when multiple frames are identified (Van Gorp, 2010). These multiple frames can also be conveyed in one message.

Throughout both codebooks, yes/no questions were used. This approach was chosen on grounds of its advantages compared to alternative options and also because it had been used productively in previous landmark framing studies (Grabe & Bucy, 2009; Semetko & Valkenburg,

2000). The main advantage of using yes/no questions is that it simplifies the coding process. The codes to be assigned do not have to be memorized or double-checked for each variable; "1" always stands for "yes," and "0" always stands for "no." Intercoder reliability coefficients can thus be expected to be high, allowing the straightforward collection of detailed and reliable data. I do acknowledge that this coding has limitations. First, the binary categories of 0 and 1 can increase the risk of measurement inaccuracies due to typos. Yet, given that acceptable intercoder reliability could be achieved, this hypothetical problem does not seem to have materialized in this study (see Coder Training, Pretest, and Coding below). Second, using the nominal level of measurement may prevent researchers from conducting certain statistical analyses that would be possible with ordinal or interval level data. Bringing the information of interest to an ordinal or interval level would have been meaningless for most variables in this study.

For each codebook, the operationalization of the framing and the sourcing variables began deductively and was continued inductively. Variables were devised first based on previous research. Correspondingly, the earliest version of the codebooks included an operationalization of all frame elements in Table 6.1 and all conceivable news sources reviewed in Chapter 4. Next, a stratified sample of 20% of the material was used to add coding examples to each variable included in this version of the codebooks. The variables for which no coding examples could be found were eliminated. Where appropriate, open variables were added instead to make sure that the corresponding information could be recorded, should it unexpectedly occur in the rest of the sample.

THE VERBAL CODEBOOK

For an individual or an institution to have been considered as a news source, that person/institution had to have been quoted—directly or indirectly—or had to have written (a portion of) the text. Quotation marks and indirect speech thus acted as cues for identifying news sources. The deductive-inductive mix of approaches revealed that the news sourcing variables could easily be grouped in the PLWHA themselves, their friends or families, other media, for-profit organizations, nonprofit organizations, medical institutions, law enforcement institutions, political institutions, art and cultural institutions, and/or individuals representing these institutions. All these potential sources were coded for each news story as either present (value = 1) or absent (value = 0). Also, coders could use an open category to record unanticipated news sources; this "other" category was rarely needed.

As for the framing variables, 17 yes/no questions were used as potential content analytical indicators of the four verbal frames. They spanned the areas suggested by previous literature and summarized in Table 6.1, namely, (1) health and fitness, (2) internal state, (3) contagion scenario, and (4) social status. As not all dimensions proposed in previous studies could be used to derive unambiguous coding categories, a few adjustments had to be made (see Table 6.4).

The variables in the first area, health and fitness, did not require any adjustment. Three yes/no questions were used to determine whether the text suggested that the PLWHA in question was in bad, average, or excellent physical health and fitness. Coders were instructed to code mentions of sickness as indicators of bad health, such as "Mejia ... struggles with side effects," "he had to go on disability," or "she developed AIDS." Average health was indicated by a more complex account of the PLWHA's health, which left the impression that, healthwise, they had good days and bad days, but the good days predominated. For instance, a PLWHA saying that she lives "a somewhat ... healthy life" was coded as having an average physical health/fitness. Finally, excellent health was signaled by reference to physically strenuous activities—such as "he is the captain of the local cycling team"—and by hyperbolic references to one's health, like "I'm in amazing shape."

The framing variables falling into the second group, internal state, could also be developed along the lines proposed by previous studies. Coders were instructed to consider a PLWHA's internal state as negative when the person seemed emotionally overwhelmed, appeared to lack

Table 6.4 Verbal Information Expected to Point to the Four Frames

	Health and Fitness	*Internal State*	*Social Status*	*Contagion Scenario*
Victim frame	Poor (symptoms, treatment, side-effects, doctor's visits)	Negative (overwhelmed, lack inner strength, negative attitude/ emotions, reduced self-determination, loneliness)	—	Drugs; sex; lifestyle and extenuating circumstances through blood, at birth, or through abuse
Survivor frame	Excellent (very healthy, sporty, health-conscious)	Excellent (great coping and inner strength, very positive; personal commitment to stop the epidemic)	—	
Carrier frame	—	—	Outcast (deviant, disease spreader)	
Normal frame	Average (good days and bad days)	Average (cope well with diagnosis)	Acceptable (like everybody else; support system)	

inner strength, and/or had a clearly negative attitude toward life—if, for instance, the individual in question was described or self-described as pessimistic, sad, hopeless, suffering from depression, having death-related thoughts, or being desperate. A PLWHA's internal state was considered average when the text suggested that the PLWHA had come to terms with the diagnosis and was generally coping well, as in "I'm HIV-positive and that's that. I've made my peace with it," or "It's hard at times, but I've been working through it." Finally, a PLWHA was considered to be in an excellent internal state when the text suggested that the individual coped better with the diagnosis than others, that he or she had a great inner strength and/or a very positive attitude toward life despite or because of the HIV status. For example, PLWHA quoted saying things like "HIV has changed my life for the better" or "For me, HIV was only the beginning of living life" were considered to suggest an excellent internal state. Unlike previous studies, this one also included a variable measuring one's personal commitment to stop the epidemic as a potential indicator of an excellent internal state. Any mention of the PLWHA being a motivational/public speaker on HIV-related topics, of activist work, or peer education was considered suggestive of such personal commitment.

By contrast, the operationalization of responsibility for the framing variables falling into the third group, contagion scenario, was quite laborious. Previous literature suggested here a clear divide between "innocent" and "guilty" PLWHA. However, most materials in the subsample used for the codebook development were very cautious about assigning blame for HIV contagion; splitting PLWHA into these two groups was virtually impossible. This was further complicated by differences in the evaluations of personal responsibility among the two coders and me. As a remedy to this problem, the coding of factual information regarding contagion (drugs, sex, lifestyle, or through blood products, at birth, or through abuse) was split from the attribution of responsibility. This was achieved by identifying whether or not the text mentioned events in the lives of the PLWHA that led them to engage in the behavior that led to their HIV infection. For instance, intravenous drug use was sometimes presented in an exculpatory fashion with reference to a major stroke of fate. While this way of extracting information from the material seemed more objective than having coders use their own moral standards to judge responsibility or guilt, it did complicate things somewhat, because it was no longer clear to which frame, if any, a given contagion scenario would belong—hence the missing values in Table 6.4.

Finally, the framing variables measuring the social status of the PLWHA were developed in accordance with previous studies. Four yes/no questions were used; through them, coders recorded whether the PLWHA were presented as reasonable, socially acceptable individuals or as vicious spreaders of disease. To be precise, a statement like "This is

Kristopher Sharp. He's running for student body vice-president. He also happens to be HIV-positive" was considered to present the PLWHA as a reasonable, socially acceptable individual. On the other hand, accounts of how unsuspecting individuals were infected because of, say, "reckless and careless behavior [...] like Mr. Davis," where Mr. Davis is an individual living with HIV/AIDS, were considered to position the PLWHA as a disease spreader. Additionally, I intended to measure whether the text suggested that the PLWHA in question had a support system or was isolated. Yet, as nothing in the subsample used for the development of the codebook suggested that PLWHA were isolated, I only kept the variable measuring the existence of a support system. Coders were instructed to code statements like "I enjoy the warm support of my family" and "they sustained me with their friendship" as suggestive of a support system. Finally, statements suggesting that the PLWHA in question was rejected by others for his or her behavior, despised, or avoided were coded as suggestive of a pariah/social-outcast status (e.g., "convicted...first-degree sex abuse and first-degree attempted unlawful sexual penetration of a 5-year-old girl".)

Table 6.4 summarizes the way the framing variables in the verbal codebook are expected to align with frames (see also Table 6.1 for comparison). Note that the extent to which each of these variables actually frame PLWHA has yet to be subjected to empirical validation.

THE VISUAL CODEBOOK

The process of devising photo sourcing variables was similar to that used for the news sources in the verbal codebook. Here, I had anticipated that the same groups acting as news sources would also act as photo sources, in addition to the newspaper or newsmagazine itself. Inductively, the list could be reduced to the following seven: the newspaper/newsmagazine; the PLWHA themselves; their friends or families; nonprofit organizations; law enforcement institutions; other media, art, and cultural institutions; and "other." For-profit organizations, medical institutions, and political institutions were not included as possible photo sources, as they did not surface in the process of codebook development.

For the visual codebook, just as for the verbal codebook, potential framing variables were developed along the lines suggested by previous studies, as summarized in Table 6.1.

Yet previous research had not attempted to extract information from visuals in a way that fully corresponded with the areas of interest for this study, namely, (1) physical fitness and health, (2) internal state, (3) contagion scenario, and (4) social status. Once again, as suggested by the missing value in Table 6.1, it is unclear how, if at all, the idea of responsibility for contracting HIV or innocence can be conveyed visually in a way that points to one frame or another (see Table 6.5).

Table 6.5 Visual Characteristics Expected to Point to the Four Frames

	Photo Content	*Nonverbal Behavior*	*Structural Features*
Victim frame	Sickness-related props	Downturned mouth corners Averted gaze Passive hands Low arms Sitting, lying, leaning Located beneath others	Camera lengths: long, medium, close-up Camera angles: high, eye-level, low
Survivor frame	Sports-related activity Sports-related props Public-address props	Upturned or relaxed mouth corners Direct gaze Hands in movement High arms Standing tall and upright Located above others	
Carrier frame	Criminality props disapproving others	Downturned or relaxed mouth corners Averted gaze Passive hands Low arms Sitting, lying, leaning	
Normal frame	Everyday activity Everyday objects or pets approving or neutral others	Upturned or relaxed mouth corners Direct gaze Hands in movement Low arms Standing tall and upright Located at the same level as others	

Thus, the task here was to determine which visual characteristics were informative in ways that corresponded with these four areas. This was a sensitive step in the codebook development, as it may be tempting to force visuals into categories adapted from the verbal codebook. To ensure that visuals were coded in a way that does justice to their characteristics (Graber, 1990; Lobinger, 2012), the codebook included questions regarding exclusively manifest content, not coders' interpretation of that content. For example, one could interpret a photo showing a person averting his or her gaze from the camera and with lowered mouth corners as one suggesting that the protagonist's internal state was negative. Yet, asking coders for such overall estimations of the internal state of the PLWHA—as positive, neutral, or negative—might be unreliable. Accordingly, coders were asked to code manifest content instead (such as direction of gaze and mouth corners' position) as this appeared more reliable.

Twenty-three yes/no questions were used to collect visual information potentially relevant to the framing of PLWHA. Coders recorded the content of the photos, nonverbal behavior, and structural features. The content-related aspects of interest regarded (a) the activity depicted, (b) the props used, and (c) others' attitudes toward the PLWHA. The (d) nonverbal behavior of the PLWHA was recorded using several micro-level variables described below. The structural features of interest were (e) camera distance and (f) camera angle. Each of these variables had several values which, according to previous research, might variably align with the four frames of interest.

Judging by previous research, two types of (a) activity were recorded on the assumption that they would be relevant to the framing of PLWHA—everyday activities and sports-related activities. Everyday activities included household chores, shopping, playing, pursuing hobbies, and so on. Sports-related activities included exercising, working out, and playing sports.

Previous research also suggested that (b) props might be consequential for the framing of PLWHA. Accordingly, the following types of props were recorded: those suggesting a public address (microphones, lecterns, etc.), those indicating illness (pills and medical equipment), those related to sports (sporting gear and sporting equipment), everyday objects and pets, and those suggesting criminality. Also, when people other than the PLWHA were shown in a photo, their (c) attitudes toward the PLWHA in question were recorded as either approving, disapproving, or neutral.

The (d) nonverbal behavior of the PLWHA depicted was recorded using the following manifest categories (see Chapter 3): mouth corners (upward, relaxed, downward), eyes (direct gaze, indirect gaze), hands (active, passive), arms (at shoulder height, lower than shoulder height), posture (standing tall or sitting, lying, hunching), and position relative to the other people depicted (beneath, same, above).

Finally, moving to the last group of variables—those concerning structural features—coders recorded (e) camera angles as either high, at eye level, or low. The (f) camera distance could be a close-up, a medium shot, a long shot, or a mug shot; the latter was added inductively as a subtype of close-ups in an attempt to identify police-made photos. The connotations of each of these visual characteristics were addressed in Chapter 3 (see Table 3.1). While previous studies on the four frames of interest here do not explicitly ascertain variations in any of these various characteristics, their inclusion in the visual codebook seemed advisable, as their connotations vary in ways that may point to some of the frames of interest (see Table 6.5). Another reason in favor of coding these aspects is that, along with nonverbal behavior, they represent genuinely visual measures. However, previous literature on the visual framing of PLWHA has only seldom investigated how various shot lengths and angles were used with certain frames; this is why the last column in Table 6.5 was merged.

Yet how do these visual characteristics fit to the four frames of interest in this study? I now address this question by referring back to the main elements of the verbal codebook: (1) health and fitness, (2) internal state, (3) contagion scenario, and (4) social status.

First, I considered that the activity in which the depicted PLWHA is engaging and the props used are informative with regard to his or her (1) health and fitness. Specifically, sports-related activity and sports-related props suggested excellent health, whereas illness-related props suggested poor health[13] (see Table 6.5).

Second, I ascertained (2) the internal state of the people depicted with reference to their nonverbal behavior (mouth corners, eyes, hands, arms, body posture, and position relative to others). Relying on previous studies,[14] I assumed that these features would align with the four frames summarized in the penultimate column in Table 6.5. Additionally, I expected that props suggesting a public address, such as a microphone, were an indicator of an excellent internal state and represented one's personal commitment to end the epidemic (see above the description of this variable for the verbal codebook). Finally, while I initially planned to operationalize loneliness (as a component of the victim frame) through photos showing PLWHA alone, this variable had to be dropped. This was due to the fact that most photos in the subsample used for codebook development showed PLWHA by themselves (while variations were noticed on the other frame elements).

Third, no variables in the visual codebook recorded the guilt or innocence of the PLWHA for (3) the contagion scenario. Several paths chosen to devise coding categories proved to be dead-ends. A first attempt was to categorize photos showing people using drugs and/or suggesting commercial sex as "guilty" and the rest as "innocent." Yet, no photos in the sample showed individuals selling sex or using drugs, so this line had to be abandoned. A second idea was to automatically categorize photos of children as "innocent," but such a variable seemed meaningless, given its redundancy with the socio-demographic question measuring age. A third pursuit involved measuring "guilt" for contagion with the help of sexualized appearance. However, as very few coding examples for this variable could be found in the subsample used for the codebook development, this last strategy also had to be discarded.

Fourth, the following visual indicators of (4) social status were devised, belonging to the domains of activity, props, and other subjects' attitude toward the PLWHA. Specifically, everyday objects and pets, everyday activities (e.g., household chores), and depictions with approving or neutral others might convey the normal frame. Conversely, the depiction of PLWHA with disapproving others might indicate that the PLWHA was an outcast (e.g., a photo showing policemen marching off a handcuffed PLWHA). Police mug shots were also deemed to be visual indicators of the outcast status of certain PLWHA (see Table 6.5).

Table 6.6 Pretest—Reliability Coefficients for Each Variable

Group	*Variable*	*α*
News sources	Does the PLWHAc or do his/her friends or family appear as news sources?	.86
	Does a for-profit enterprise/company or individual/s representing it appear as news sources?	.90
	Does a nonprofit organization or individual/s representing it appear as news sources?	.90
	Does a medical institution or individual/s representing it appear as a news source?	.87
	Does a law enforcement institution or individual/s representing it appear as a news source?	1.0
	Do other media or individual/s representing them appear as news sources?	.85
	Does a federal or local agency/political institution or individual/s representing it appear/s as a news source?	.84
	Do individual/s representing the culture, leisure, and entertainment industries appear as news sources?	.87
	Is someone else appearing as a news source? [string]	.96
Socio-demographic characteristics of the PLWHA	What gender is the PLWHAc? Male	1.0
	What gender is the PLWHAc? Female	1.0
	What sexuality is the PLWHAc? Heterosexual	.97
	What sexuality is the PLWHAc? Homosexual	1.0
	What sexuality is the PLWHAc? Bisexual	.90
Health and internal state	Does the text suggest that the PLWHAc is in (somewhat) bad physical health and fitness?	.87
	Does the text suggest that the PLWHAc is in average health?	.92
	Does the text suggest that the PLWHAc is in excellent physical health and fitness?	1.0
	Does the text suggest that the PLWHAc is emotionally overwhelmed, lacks inner strength, or has a clearly negative attitude toward life?	.87
	Does the text suggest that the PLWHAc has come to terms with the diagnosis and generally copes well with it?	.93
	Does the text suggest that the PLWHAc is coping better than others with the diagnosis, has great inner strength, or has a very positive attitude toward life?	1.0
	Does the text suggest that the PLWHAc is a motivational/public speaker, activist, peer educator, or is volunteering at an HIV/AIDS charity or organization?	.95
Contagion scenario	Does the text suggest that the PLWHAc contracted HIV through drug use?	.85
	Does the text suggest that the PLWHAc contracted HIV through commercial sex?	1.0

Group	Variable	α
	Does the text suggest that the PLWHAc contracted HIV through noncommercial sex?	.96
	Does the text suggest that the PLWHAc contracted HIV through contaminated blood products, at birth, or through abuse?	1.0
	Does the text suggest that the PLWHAc contracted HIV as a result of their behavior or lifestyle?	1.0
	Does the text include any mention of extenuating circumstances regarding the contagion scenario?	.97
Social status	Does the text suggest that the people in the life of the PLWHAc are supportive?	.83
	Does the text suggest that the PLWHA is a reasonable, socially acceptable individual?	.81
	Does the text suggest that the PLWHAc infected other people on purpose?	1.0
	Does the text suggest that the PLWHAc is a pariah or an outcast?	.85
Photo sources	Is the medium publishing the photo or an individual photographer named as a photo source?	.98
	Is the PLWHAc or his/her friends or family named as a photo source?	.88
	Is a nonprofit organization or individual/s representing it named as a photo source?	.90
	Is a law enforcement institution or an individual representing it named as a photo source?	1.0
	Is another medium or individual/s representing them appear as photo sources?	.97
	Are individuals representing the culture, leisure, and entertainment industries named as photo sources?	1.0
	Is someone else named as a photo source?	1.0
Structural features	Is this a close-up?	1.0
	If the photo is a close-up, is it also a mug shot?	1.0
	Is this a medium shot?	.97
	Is this a long shot?	.96
	Is this a high-angle shot?	.92
	Is this a low-angle shot?	.94
	Is this an eye-level shot?	.96
Socio-demographic characteristics	Is the PLWHAc up to 12 years old?	1.0
	Is the PLWHAc a teenager (13–19 years old)?	.96
	Is the PLWHAc an adult (20–49 years old)?	.90
	Is the PLWHAc 50 years old or older?	.88
	Is the PLWHAc white?	.97
	Is the PLWHAc Hispanic/Latino?	.91
	Is the PLWHAc black/African American?	1.0
	Is the PLWHAc Asian/Asian American?	1.0
	Is the race/ethnicity of the PLWHAc none of the above, or you can't tell which one it is?	1.0

(*Continued*)

Group	*Variable*	*α*
Activity, props, other subjects	Is the PLWHAc shown exercising, working out, playing sports?	1.0
	Is the PLWHAc shown doing household chores, shopping, playing, dancing, or pursuing hobbies other than sports?	.92
	Are pills or medical equipment visible in the photo?	1.0
	Is sporting gear or equipment visible in the photo?	1.0
	Is a microphone, banner, podium, lectern, stage, or a photo op wall visible in the photo?	1.0
	Are everyday objects or pets visible in the photo?	.96
	Are objects suggesting criminality visible in the photo?	1.0
	If the PLWHAc is depicted with other people, do others' gestures, posture, or facial expressions suggest that they approve of the PLWHAc?	.96
	If the PLWHAc is depicted with other people, do others' gestures, posture, or facial expressions suggest that they neither approve nor disapprove of the PLWHAc?	.94
	If the PLWHAc is depicted with other people, do others' gestures, posture, or facial expressions suggest that they disapprove of the PLWHAc?	1.0
Nonverbal behavior	Are the mouth corners of the PLWHAc upturned?	.95
	Are the mouth corners of the PLWHAc neither upturned nor downturned?	.94
	Are the mouth corners of the PLWHAc downturned?	1.0
	Is the PLWHAc looking directly at the camera or someone?	.89
	Are the eyes of the PLWHAc looking indirectly, up or down, or are they closed?	.92
	Are the hands of the PLWHAc depicted in movement?	.94
	Are the hands of the PLWHAc at rest, passive?	.95
	Is at least one arm of the PLWHAc held at shoulder height?	.89
	Are the arms of the PLWHAc located lower than shoulder height?	.95
	Is the PLWHAc standing tall and upright?	.97
	Is the PLWHAc sitting, lying, or leaning (backward, forward, or to the side), or is s/he hunched over, bowed, or slumped?	.96
	If the PLWHAc is depicted with other people, is the PLWHAc located beneath others?	1.0
	If the PLWHAc is depicted with other people, are they located at the same level?	.94
	If the PLWHAc is depicted with other people, is the PLWHAc located above the rest?	.86

Note: PLWHAc = PLWHA to whom the coding referred.

Coder Training, Pretest, and Coding

Three German undergraduate students were involved in the pretest and data collection for this study. One took part in the coding of both words and photos (conducted separately); the other two were involved in just the word or the photo coding. This resulted in two teams of two coders each for the word coding and the photo coding, respectively.

Several weeks were necessary for the testing of categories and coder training. During this time, various refinements were made to the codebooks. The articles used during these coding sessions were included in the final sample. Before the actual coding began and the sample was split among the coders, one final pretest on a stratified 20% of the sample was conducted. Intercoder reliability was measured using Krippendorff's alpha in SPSS, where values above .80 represent strong reliability (Hayes & Krippendorff, 2007). Scores were between .81 and 1.0 for each variable in the final pretest (see Table 6.6). Once the training and pretest were completed, coders started coding independently. The verbal sample was coded first; the visual sample was coded second.[15]

Efforts were made to keep coder subjectivity and coder bias to a minimum to increase validity and reliability. First, to ensure that the coding of the verbal component of the material was not influenced by the information contained in the visuals and vice versa, the word coding and the photo coding were conducted separately (see Figure 5.1). Second, clear-cut manifest coding categories were used. For instance, coders were asked to distinguish between particular hands, arms, and eye movements of the PLWHA; they were not asked to rate whether nonverbal behaviors belonged to the normal, carrier, survivor, or victim frames. The assignment of manifest variables to latent constructs—the frames—was carried out during data analysis.

Results

Frame Identification

As mentioned above, the frames of interest in this study were encountered in previous literature. The codebooks used to collect data from the verbal and the visual sample, respectively, consisted mainly of variables operationalizing the frame definitions proposed toward the beginning of this chapter following a thorough review of previous studies.

As frames were not coded holistically but were instead divided into several elements that were coded individually, reliability analyses in SPSS were needed to test whether the variables devised to measure frame elements occurred together as summarized in Tables 6.4 and 6.5, respectively.

Provided these analyses return Cronbach's alphas above .6 (Hair, Black, Babin, Anderson, & Tatham, 2006), the respective variables were indexed together. These indexes helped identify the frames and their respective weight in the material. To achieve this, the total number of frame elements in a particular instance was divided by the maximum number of frame elements for that particular frame. Thus, the scores indicated values ranging from .00 (frame not present) to 1.00 (frame present): the closer the value to 1.00, the higher the number of frame elements that were encountered, and thus the higher the weight of that frame. For example, when the Cronbach's alpha suggested there were four elements to the normal frame, but only three of them were encountered in the newspaper article at hand, the value recorded in the index was .75. Recording a frame's weight was deemed important, as this allowed the identification of the dominant frame for each PLWHA in the sample, not just whether or not that frame occurs (see Chapter 3; Matthes, 2007; Van Gorp, 2010).

Verbal Frames

According to previous studies, PLWHA presented through the victim frame appear to be in poor health and fitness, and their internal state is presented as negative (see Table 6.4). Submitting the two variables measuring these aspects to a reliability analysis indicated marginally acceptable internal consistency (Cronbach's $\alpha = .65$).

Previous studies suggested that when a survivor frame is used for the presentation of PLWHA, the individuals in question appeared not just to be in excellent health and fitness but also to have an excellent inner state. The latter is denoted by great coping with the diagnosis on the one hand and a personal commitment to stop the epidemic on the other hand. The reliability analysis revealed marginally acceptable internal consistency for these three variables ($\alpha = .68$).

Earlier studies proposed that when PLWHA are presented through the carrier frame, they appear as disease spreaders and outcasts. The reliability analysis revealed an acceptable internal consistency when these two variables were combined (Cronbach's $\alpha = .78$).

Finally, previous literature suggested that when PLWHA are presented through the normal frame, their internal state and their health and fitness are presented as average. Moreover, they appear like everybody else and have a support system. The four variables measuring these aspects were submitted to a reliability analysis in SPSS. The Cronbach's alpha indicated good internal consistency ($\alpha = .83$).

Above, I explained why the way PLWHA contracted HIV may or may not contribute to the framing of PLWHA. This possibility was tested by conducting reliability analyses between the variables listed above for each of the four frames and the variables recording the specific contagion scenario (e.g., drugs) and whether or not the contagion scenario was presented in an exculpatory way. This was done by adding one variable at the time, all variables at once, and one aggregate variable (contagion scenario mentioned? yes/no) to the reliability analysis. Without exception, each of these efforts led to a serious deterioration of the alpha value for each frame (on average to .40). Thus, it seemed that the way PLWHA contracted HIV no longer qualifies as a key component of any of the four frames investigated in this study.

Visual Frames

Earlier studies suggested that PLWHA depicted through the victim frame are shown with sickness-related props and exhibit negative nonverbal behavior (see Table 6.5). Yet in this study, submitting the two variables[16] measuring these aspects to a reliability analysis in SPSS suggested otherwise. The Cronbach's alpha indicated unacceptable internal consistency ($\alpha = .09$). Similarly low alphas were obtained when the variable recoding sickness-related props was submitted to a reliability analysis with each of the variables recoding camera angle and camera distance. Thus, only the variable recording sickness-related props was kept as an indicator of the victim frame.

As shown in Table 6.5, previous literature suggested that PLWHA depicted through the survivor frame are portrayed engaging in a sports-related activity, with sports-related and/or public-address props. Also, these PLWHA may be shown exhibiting positive nonverbal behavior. Finally, there is a possibility that certain camera angles and camera distances are used preferentially. All these variables were submitted to the reliability analysis in every conceivable combination. An acceptable internal consistency was obtained only when combining the variable measuring sports-related activity and that recording the presence of sports-related props (Cronbach's $\alpha = .90$).

Previous studies have proposed that the carrier frame can be conveyed visually when PLWHA are depicted together with criminality props, disapproving others, and negative nonverbal behavior. There was also a possibility that camera angles and camera distances contributed to the articulation of this visual frame (see Table 6.5). Again, all variables shown in Table 6.5 for the carrier frame were submitted to the reliability analysis in every conceivable combination. The analysis returned acceptable alphas for the following three variables: criminality props, disapproving others, and police mug shot (Cronbach's $\alpha = .74$).

Earlier studies revealed that—when they are depicted through the normal frame—PLWHA are shown engaging in an everyday activity, using everyday objects, in the company of pets, and with approving/neutral others (see Table 6.5). They may also exhibit neutral-to-positive nonverbal behavior, and certain camera angles and distances may be preferred. The only combination of variables submitted to the reliability analysis that obtained an acceptable alpha were those recording portrayals of everyday activities and approving others (Cronbach's $\alpha = .79$).

Interim Summary

Some differences were noticed between the way the four frames of interest were operationalized in previous studies and the way they surfaced in the sample used in this study. One notable difference regards the role played by the way the PLWHA in question contracted HIV. In my sample, the various contagion scenarios did not align variably with the four frames. Another difference worth mentioning concerns the type of visual information relevant to the visual framing of PLWHA. With one exception—police mug shots for the carrier frame—nonverbal behavior and structural features did not qualify as frame elements. Only photo content was relevant for the visual frames. This circumstance had been anticipated and led to the proposal of hypotheses and research questions specific to the way, if at all, nonverbal behavior and structural features nonetheless aligned with the four frames (see Chapter 6).

Tables 6.7 and 6.8 summarize the elements of the four frames of interest, both in their verbal (Table 6.7) and visual expression (Table 6.8). With the identification of the frames, the penultimate step of the integrative framing analysis is complete (see Figure 5.1). To reiterate, Step 5a concerned the identification of verbal frames, whereas Step 5b regarded the identification of visual frames. The variables resulting from this procedure were used to address the research questions and hypotheses proposed.

Descriptives

The verbal ($n = 656$) and visual ($n = 580$) framing of people living with HIV/AIDS (PLWHA) was analyzed in news, special-interest/niche publications (SIPs), and public service announcements (PSAs).

Table 6.7 Verbal Frames and Their Elements

	Health and Fitness	*Internal State*	*Social Status*
Victim frame	Poor	Negative	—
Survivor frame	Excellent	Excellent (great coping; activism)	—
Carrier frame	—	—	Outcast (outcast; disease spreader)
Normal frame	Average	Average	Acceptable (like everybody else; support system)

Table 6.8 Visual Frames and Their Elements

	Photo Content	*Nonverbal Behavior*	*Structural Features*
Victim frame	Sickness-related props	—	—
Survivor frame	Sports-related activity Sports-related props	—	—
Carrier frame	Criminality props Disapproving others	—	Police mug shot
Normal frame	Everyday activity Approving others	—	—

In the news articles, more than two thirds of the PLWHA were male (71.1%), almost all were adults (95.1%), over half were white (59.8%), and little more than a quarter were heterosexual (27.3%); almost as many were homosexual (26.9%). A third of the PLWHA in news were African American/black (33.3%); 5.4% were Hispanics/Latinos.

In PSAs, 57.3% of the PLWHA were male, 33% were heterosexual, and 13.6% were homosexual. Furthermore, 87% were adult. Most were African Americans/black (45.2%), followed by whites (38.4%) and Hispanics/Latinos (14.4%).

In SIPs, most PLWHA were male (71.1%) and homosexual (26.4%); 15.4% were heterosexual. The PLWHA shown here were almost exclusively adults (99.6%). The largest racial/ethnic group in this subsample was African American/black (40.9%), followed by white (38.3%) and Hispanic/Latino (17.4%).

The Framing of PLWHA

Variations by Communication Context and Frame Building

H1a predicted that the victim and the carrier frames would be used significantly more in news than in SIPs and PSAs; H1b projected that the normal and the survivor frames would be conveyed significantly more in SIPs and PSAs than in news. For each modality (verbal, visual), these hypotheses were tested by crosstabbing two variables: one recording the frames (normal, survivor, victim, carrier) and one the communication context (news, SIPs, PSAs). A Chi-square test revealed significant differences in the way the verbal expression of the frames (χ^2 (6) = 202.905, $p < .001$, Cramér's V = .434) was used in each communication context. Significant differences were also observed in the way the visual expression of the frames was used in each communication context (χ^2 (6) = 83.436, $p < .001$, Cramér's V = .400).

H1a was partly supported. The victim frame was conveyed for 17.4% of the PLWHA featured in news texts, which is significantly more than in SIPs (4.0%) and PSAs (3.0%). The verbal carrier frame was conveyed for 24.8% of the PLWHA in news, significantly more than for those in SIPs (0.4%) and PSAs (3.0%) (see Table 6.9). No significant differences were noticed in the way the visual victim and carrier frames were used in each communication context (see Table 6.10).

Partial support was found for H1b. The verbal normal frame was encountered significantly more in PSAs (62.0%) than in SIPs (20.5%) and news (31.7%). Also, as predicted, the verbal survivor frame was used significantly more in SIPs (75.2%) than in news (26.1%). However, no statistically significant difference between news and PSAs was observed with regard to their use of the survivor frame (see Table 6.9). As for their visual expression, the normal frame was encountered significantly more in PSA photos (94.6%) and SIPs photos (89.2%) than in news photos (43.8%)—as anticipated. However, contrary to my prediction, the visual survivor frame was used significantly more in news (27.7%) than in both SIPs (2.7%) and PSAs (5.4%) (see Table 6.10).

Table 6.9 Chi-Square Test of Significance for Verbal Frames and Communication Context (News, SIPs, and PSAs)

	News		*SIPs*		*PSAs*	
Frames	*Count*	*%*	*Count*	*%*	*Count*	*%*
Normal	51	31.7_a***	57	20.5_b***	62	62.0_c***
Survivor	42	26.1_a	209	75.2_b***	32	32.0_a
Victim	28	17.4_a***	11	4.0_b	3	3.0_b
Carrier	40	24.8_a***	1	0.4_b	3	3.0_b

Notes: * $p < .05$ ** $p < .01$ *** $p < .001$. Subscript letters indicate pairs that are significantly different (Bonferroni correction).

Table 6.10 Chi-Square Test of Significance for Visual Frames and Communication Context (News, SIPs, and PSAs)

	News		*SIPs*		*PSAs*	
Frames	*Count*	*%*	*Count*	*%*	*Count*	*%*
Normal	49	43.8_a***	33	89.2_b	106	94.6_b
Survivor	31	27.7_a***	1	2.7_b	6	5.4_b
Victim	12	10.7_a	3	8.1_a	0	0
Carrier	20	17.9_a	0	0	0	0

Note: * $p < .05$ ** $p < .01$ *** $p < .001$. Subscript letters indicate pairs that are significantly different (Bonferroni correction).

As a general observation, the verbal expression of all frames of interest appeared across all communication contexts investigated (see Table 6.9). However, this was not the case for their visual expression: all four frames were encountered in news, but just three in SIP and only two in PSAs (see Table 6.10). Also, overall, the survivor, carrier, and victim frames were conveyed significantly more verbally than visually, whereas the opposite was the case for the normal frame, which was conveyed significantly more visually than verbally (χ^2 (3) = 45.774, $p < .001$, Cramér's V = .243; results not tabled).

H2 predicted that the verbal and visual frames conveyed in a news article would differ significantly among the news sources and photo sources used. H2a investigated differences in the use of verbal frames; H2b examined differences in the use of visual frames. These hypotheses were addressed using a Chi-square test of significance and a Fisher's Exact Test, respectively, with a Bonferroni correction on a subsample of the material, which recorded the framing of PLWHA in news articles (n = 242) and in news photos (n = 204). The data set was restructured from a wide format (i.e., where all news/photo sources used in an article were listed in one row) to a long format (i.e., where at most one news/photo source was listed in each row).

For H2a, the procedure consisted of crosstabs between a variable recording the verbal frames (normal, survivor, victim, carrier) and a variable recording the news sources (PLWHA, their friends or family, nonprofits, law enforcement, medical and research institutions, other sources). "News sources" refers to organizations or individuals that offered journalists the information used in the article. The most frequent news sources in sample were PLWHA, their friends, or family (72.7%); nonprofits (42.6%); law enforcement (28.9%); medical and research institutions (17.4%); and representatives of the art and leisure sector (16.1%). For-profits (13.2%), other media (12%), politics (10.3%), and other (string; 3.7%) were the least common sources. The percentages exceed 100 because more than one news source per article could be coded. For the analysis, for-profits, other media, political institutions, and other were collapsed into one category labeled "other," because only few observations were recorded for each of them.

As predicted by H2a, the verbal frames conveyed in news differed significantly among the news sources used, χ^2 (12) = 105.090, $p < .001$, Cramér's V = .317. As shown in Table 6.11, the normal frame was used significantly more when PLWHA, their friends and family (36.2%), nonprofit organizations (39.1%), and medical institutions (40.6%) were used as news sources than when journalists used news sources from law enforcement (2.8%). Similarly, the survivor frame was used significantly more when PLWHA, their friends and family (27.6%), nonprofit organizations (28.1%), and other sources (32.2%) were used as news sources than when journalists used news sources from law enforcement (2.8%). No significant differences were observed for the use of the verbal victim frame. Finally, the verbal carrier frame was used significantly more when law enforcement news sources were used (88.9%) than when any other type of sources was used, namely, PLWHA, their friends and family (16.5%), nonprofit organizations (10.9%), medical and research institutions (18.8%), and other (13.3%; see Table 6.11).

Analogous to the procedure for H2a, a crosstab between a variable recording the visual frames (normal, survivor, victim, carrier) and a variable recording the photo sources (media, other) was used to test H2b. The term "photo sources" denotes the organizations or individuals that provided the visuals selected to illustrate the news article. For this study, the following frequencies were observed: the newspaper itself (51.5%); other media (27.9%); law enforcement institutions (4.9%); PLWHA, family, or friends (4.4%); nonprofit organizations (1.5%); art/leisure (0.5%); and other photo sources (string; 0.5%). Due to the scarce occurrence of photo sources other than media-based ones, the photo sources in this study were collapsed into just two groups: one was labeled "media" (the newspaper itself and other media); one was labeled "other" (the other five photo sources).

As predicted by H2b, the visual frames conveyed in news differed significantly among the photo sources used, Fisher's Exact Test = 31.706, $p < .001$, Cramér's V = .691 (see Table 6.12). The visual carrier frame was conveyed significantly more often when photo sources outside the media provided the photo (69.2% vs. 3.4%). A more in-depth look at the data revealed that nine of the 12 photos in which a visual carrier frame was conveyed were mug shots provided by law enforcement. No other significant paired comparisons were found (see Table 6.12).

Variations by Medium Characteristics and/or Communication Goals

H3a and H3b anticipated that the frames would be used differently in news based on the structure of the community in which the newspapers were published. These hypotheses were tested using the crosstabs procedure between a variable recording the verbal frames or the visual frames, respectively (normal, survivor, victim, carrier), and variables recording conservatism (high/low), urbanism (high/low), religiosity (high/low), and HIV/AIDS prevalence in the region (high/low).

In order to test these hypotheses, survey data and CDC statistics were consulted and included in the analysis. First, Gallup data were used to

Table 6.11 Chi-Square Test of Significance for Verbal News Frames and News Sources

	News Sources									
	PLWHA, Friends or Family		*Nonprofit Organizations*		*Law Enforcement*		*Medical and Research Institutions*		*Other*	
Verbal News Frames	*Count*	%	*Count*	%	*Count*	%	*Count*	%	*Count*	%
Normal	46	36.2_a	25	39.1_a	1	2.8_b***	13	40.6_a	31	34.4_a
Survivor	35	27.6_a	18	28.1_a	1	2.8_b***	8	$25.0_{a,b}$	29	32.2_a
Victim	25	19.7_a	14	21.9_a	2	5.6_a	5	15.6_a	18	20.0_a
Carrier	21	16.5_a	7	10.9_a	32	88.9_b***	6	18.8_a	12	13.3_a

Note: * $p < .05$ ** $p < .01$ *** $p < .001$. Subscript letters indicate pairs that are significantly different (Bonferroni correction).

Table 6.12 Fisher's Exact Test for Visual News Frames and Photo Sources

	Photo Sources			
	Media		*Other*	
Visual News Frames	*Count*	*%*	*Count*	*%*
Normal	45	50.6_a	4	30.8_a
Survivor	29	32.6_a	0	
Victim	12	13.5_a	0	
Carrier	3	3.4_a	9	69.2_b***

Note: * $p < .05$ ** $p < .01$ *** $p < .001$. Subscript letters indicate pairs that are significantly different (Bonferroni correction).

categorize news texts and news photos as coming from newspapers published in states scoring high or low on conservatism, urbanism, and religiosity. For conservatism, the concept of conservative advantage was used to split the sample in two groups. Conservative advantage refers to "the percentage of residents self-identifying as conservative minus the percentage self-identifying as liberal in each state" (Swift, 2014). Conservatism was considered high when the conservative advantage was ≥5% and as low when it was <5%; see Table 6.13. For urbanism, the division was made at 90%, where high urbanism was set ≥90%, and low urbanism at <90% (see Table 6.14). The percentage of those very religious was used to identify groups of high and low for religiosity: ≥35% (high) and <35% (low); see Table 6.15. Finally, CDC data were used to distinguish between newspapers published in states with high or low HIV/AIDS rates: HIV rates per 100,000 ≥ 10 (high); HIV rates per 100,000 < 10 (low); see Table 6.16.

As shown in Table 6.17, there were statistically significant differences in the occurrence of verbal frames in news articles by the characteristics of the state—that is, conservatism (χ^2 (3) = 40.229, $p < .001$, Cramér's V = .508), urbanism (χ^2 (3) = 9.750, $p < .05$, Cramér's V = .250), religiosity (χ^2 (3) = 42.584, $p < .001$, Cramér's V = .522), and HIV/AIDS prevalence (χ^2 (3) = 19.219, $p < .001$, Cramér's V = .351). As for the visual frames, statistically significant differences were only observed between the visual frames and HIV/AIDS prevalence (χ^2 (3) = 11.953, $p < .05$, Cramér's V = .328), but not religiosity (χ^2 (3) = 3.340, $p = .34$), conservatism (χ^2 (3) = 5.400, $p = .14$), or urbanism (Fisher's Exact Test = 3.936, $p = .25$); see Table 6.18.

H3a predicted that the normal, survivor, and victim frames would be used significantly more in news from states characterized by low conservatism, low religiosity, high HIV/AIDS prevalence, and high urbanism than in their counterparts. This hypothesis was partly supported. As shown in Table 6.17, the verbal normal frame was used significantly more in news from states sharing three of the four characteristics predicted. Specifically, it was used significantly more in newspapers issued in states

Table 6.13 News Sites in Sample by Political Views in the State

State	*News Site in Sample*	*% Conservative*	*% Moderate*	*% Liberal*	*Conservative Advantage*
District of Columbia	*Washington Post*	21.6	35.4	38.1	–16.5
New York	*New York Post*	29.4	35.8	27.6	1.8
New York	*New York Times*	29.4	35.8	27.6	1.8
California	*Los Angeles Times*	30.2	36.5	27.5	2.7
New Jersey	*Newark Star-Ledger*	29.9	37.8	25.5	4.4
Oregon	*The Oregonian*	33.8	33.7	27.5	6.3
Illinois	*Chicago Sun-Times*	31.6	37.7	24.6	7.0
Minnesota	*Star Tribune*	34.7	36.0	24.4	10.3
Arizona	*The Arizona Republic*	36.1	36.1	22.3	13.8
Wisconsin	*Milwaukee Journal Sentinel*	36.4	36.7	21.5	14.9
Florida	*Tampa Bay Times*	36.6	35.7	21.7	14.9
Ohio	*Plain Dealer*	36.9	37.3	20.8	16.1
North Carolina	*Charlotte Observer*	38.9	33.9	21.5	17.4
Kansas	*The Wichita Eagle*	38.4	36.3	20.4	18.0
Texas	*Dallas Morning News*	39.9	34.9	19.0	20.9
Missouri	*St. Louis Post-Dispatch*	39.8	36.5	18.4	21.4
Montana	*Missoulian*	43.1	31.7	21.1	22.0
Kentucky	*The Courier-Journal*	41.8	33.8	18.2	23.6
Tennessee	*The Tennessean*	43.2	34.0	16.8	26.4
Utah	*The Salt-Lake Tribune*	44.6	34.1	17.4	27.2
Arkansas	*Arkansas Democrat Gazette*	43.8	33.0	16.4	27.4
Alabama	*Montgomery Advertiser*	46.5	31.3	15.3	31.2

Sources: Gallup (2014) and Swift (2014).

Table 6.14 News Sites in Sample Ranked by Rural-Urban Ratio in the State

State	*News Site*	*Percentage of the Total Population of the State Represented by the Urban Population*
District of Columbia	*Washington Post*	100
California	*Los Angeles Times*	94.95
New Jersey	*Newark Star-Ledger*	94.68
Florida	*Tampa Bay Times*	91.16
Utah	*The Salt-Lake Tribune*	90.58
Arizona	*The Arizona Republic*	89.81
Illinois	*Chicago Sun-Times*	88.49
New York	*New York Post*	87.87
New York	*New York Times*	87.87
Texas	*Dallas Morning News*	84.7
Oregon	*The Oregonian*	81.03
Ohio	*Plain Dealer*	77.92
Kansas	*The Wichita Eagle*	74.2
Minnesota	*Star Tribune*	73.27
Missouri	*St. Louis Post-Dispatch*	70.44
Wisconsin	*Milwaukee Journal Sentinel*	70.15
Tennessee	*The Tennessean*	66.39
North Carolina	*Charlotte Observer*	66.09
Alabama	*Montgomery Advertiser*	59.04
Kentucky	*The Courier-Journal*	58.38
Arkansas	*Arkansas Democrat Gazette*	56.16
Montana	*Missoulian*	55.89

Source: United States Census Bureau (2014).

characterized by low conservatism (43.4%), low religiosity (42.3%), and high HIV/AIDS prevalence (36.7%) than in their counterparts (see Table 6.17). Significant differences in the predicted direction were also observed with the verbal survivor frame, which was conveyed significantly more in newspapers from states with high urbanism (40.5%) than in those from states scoring low on urbanism (20.2%). Also, the victim frame was encountered significantly more in news outlets exhibiting two of the four prognosticated characteristics: low conservatism (26.3%) and low religiosity (26.9%).

As seen in Table 6.18, statistically significant differences were observed between the visual frames and HIV/AIDS prevalence. Specifically, the visual survivor frame was conveyed more in newspapers from states with high HIV rates (34.2%) than in their counterparts (11.4%). Contrary to my prediction, the visual victim frame was conveyed more often in news outlets from states with low HIV rates (20%) than in their counterparts (6.6%). No significant differences were noticed for the normal frame (see Table 6.18). Contrary to my prediction, no significant difference in the visual framing of PLWHA was observed based on religiosity, conservatism, and urbanism.

Table 6.15 News Sites in Sample by Religiosity in the State

State	*News Site in Sample*	*% Very Religious*	*% Moderately Religious*	*% Nonreligious*
Oregon	*The Oregonian*	29.3	27.2	43.4
District of Columbia	*Washington Post*	30.0	29.0	41.0
New York	*New York Post*	32.7	30.3	37.1
New York	*New York Times*	32.7	30.3	37.1
California	*Los Angeles Times*	33.6	28.6	37.8
Montana	*Missoulian*	35.0	27.2	37.8
New Jersey	*Newark Star-Ledger*	35.6	31.8	32.5
Arizona	*The Arizona Republic*	37.7	28.5	33.8
Florida	*Tampa Bay Times*	38.2	31.0	30.8
Wisconsin	*Milwaukee Journal Sentinel*	38.5	28.8	32.7
Illinois	*Chicago Sun-Times*	38.6	28.7	32.6
Ohio	*Plain Dealer*	38.8	30.2	31.0
Minnesota	*Star Tribune*	39.5	26.4	34.2
Kansas	*The Wichita Eagle*	40.7	28.7	30.6
Missouri	*St. Louis Post-Dispatch*	42.7	30.0	27.3
Texas	*Dallas Morning News*	47.7	30.8	21.5
Kentucky	*The Courier-Journal*	48.7	29.0	22.3
North Carolina	*Charlotte Observer*	50.2	30.2	19.6
Tennessee	*The Tennessean*	51.0	30.9	18.2
Arkansas	*Arkansas Democrat Gazette*	54.6	27.8	17.6
Alabama	*Montgomery Advertiser*	57.6	28.8	13.6
Utah	*The Salt-Lake Tribune*	57.6	15.2	27.2

Sources: Gallup (2014) and Newport (2013).

Table 6.16 News Sites in Sample by HIV/AIDS Prevalence in the State

State	*News Site in Sample*	*HIV Rates per 100,000 Population*
Montana	*Missoulian*	2.2
Utah	*The Salt-Lake Tribune*	3.3
Wisconsin	*Milwaukee Journal Sentinel*	4.8
Kansas	*The Wichita Eagle*	5.2
Minnesota	*Star Tribune*	6.0
Oregon	*The Oregonian*	6.7
Kentucky	*The Courier-Journal*	7.9
Arkansas	*Arkansas Democrat Gazette*	8.3
Missouri	*St. Louis Post-Dispatch*	9.4
Ohio	*Plain Dealer*	10.6
Arizona	*The Arizona Republic*	10.9
Tennessee	*The Tennessean*	14.5
California	*Los Angeles Times*	15.8
Illinois	*Chicago Sun-Times*	16.6
North Carolina	*Charlotte Observer*	17.3
Alabama	*Montgomery Advertiser*	17.6
New Jersey	*Newark Star-Ledger*	17.8
Texas	*Dallas Morning News*	19.7
New York	*New York Post*	25.5
New York	*New York Times*	25.5
Florida	*Tampa Bay Times*	28.4
District of Columbia	*Washington Post*	155.6

Source: CDC (2013c).

H3b proposed that the carrier frame would be used significantly more in news from states characterized by high conservatism, high religiosity, low HIV/AIDS prevalence, and low urbanism than in their counterparts. This hypothesis was supported.

As shown in Table 6.17, the verbal carrier frame was significantly more common in newspapers published in states sharing the following characteristics than in their counterparts: high conservatism (46.3%), low urbanism (30.3%), high religiosity (47.4%), and low HIV/AIDS prevalence (52.8%). In the visual sample, statistically significant differences were only noticed with regard to the prevalence of HIV/AIDS, in that the carrier frame was encountered significantly more in the coverage from states with low HIV rates (28.6%) than in their counterparts (13.2%) (see Table 6.18).

H4 predicted that the normal and the survivor frames would be used significantly more in SIPs targeted at PLWHA than in those directed at other subpopulations. To test this hypothesis, the variables recording the frames (verbal, visual) were crosstabbed with those recording the

Table 6.17 Chi-Square Test of Significance for Verbal News Frames and State Characteristics

	Conservatism				*Urbanism*				*Religiosity*				*HIV/AIDS Prevalence*			
	High		*Low*		*High*		*Low*		*High*		*Low*		*High*		*Low*	
Frames	*Count*	%	*Count*	%	*Count*	%	*Count*	%	*Count*	%	*Count*	%	*Count*	%	*Count*	%
Normal	17	21.3_a***	33	43.4_b***	10	27.0_a	40	33.6_a	17	21.8_a***	33	42.3_b***	44	36.7_a***	6	16.7_b***
Survivor	19	23.8_a	20	26.3_a	15	40.5_a*	24	20.2_b*	18	23.1_a	21	26.9_a	34	28.3_a	5	13.9_a
Victim	7	8.8_a***	20	26.3_b***	8	21.6_a	19	16.0_a	6	7.7_a***	21	26.9_b***	21	17.5_a	6	16.7_a
Carrier	37	46.3_a***	3	3.9_b***	4	10.8_a*	36	30.3_b*	37	47.4_a***	3	3.8_b***	21	17.5_a***	19	52.8_b***

Note: * $p < .05$ ** $p < .01$ *** $p < .001$. Subscript letters indicate pairs that are significantly different (Bonferroni correction).

Table 6.18 Chi-Square Test of Significance/Fisher's Exact Test for Visual News Frames and State Characteristics

	Conservatism				*Urbanism*				*Religiosity*				*HIV/AIDS Prevalence*			
	High		*Low*		*High*		*Low*		*High*		*Low*		*High*		*Low*	
Frames	*Count*	%	*Count*	%	*Count*	%	*Count*	%	*Count*	%	*Count*	%	*Count*	%	*Count*	%
Normal	28	38.9_a	21	53.8_a	8	53.3_a	41	42.7_a	27	39.1_a	22	52.4_a	35	46.1_a	14	40.0_a
Survivor	18	25.0_a	12	30.8_a	6	40.0_a	24	25.0_a	18	26.1_a	12	28.6_a	26	34.2_a	4	11.4_b*
Victim	10	13.9_a	2	5.1_a	0		12	12.5_a	9	13.0_a	3	7.1_a	5	6.6_a	7	20.0_b*
Carrier	16	22.2_a	4	10.3_a	1	6.7_a	19	19.8_a	15	21.7_a	5	11.9_a	10	13.2_a	10	28.6_b*

Note: * $p < .05$ ** $p < .01$ *** $p < .001$. Subscript letters indicate pairs that are significantly different (Bonferroni correction).

target audience of SIPs (PLWHA vs. African Americans and LGBT). This hypothesis had to be rejected, as there were no significant differences in framing by the target audience of the SIPs, neither for verbal frames (Fisher's Exact Test = 6.012, p = .09) nor for visual frames (Fisher's Exact Test = 2.037, p = .70). As seen in Table 6.19, about 70% of the verbal frames in SIPs were survivor frames, regardless of the target audience. Alternatively, as summarized in Table 6.20, about 80% of the visual frames were normal frames, notwithstanding the target audience. From this perspective, it is not surprising that the small differences in proportions identified in the sample were not statistically significant.

RQ1 asked if frames conveyed in PSAs differed significantly based on the type of PSA. To address this research question, the variable recording the frames (verbal, visual) was crosstabbed with the one recording the PSA type (prevention vs. treatment and anti-stigma). Significant differences were found for the verbal frames (Fisher's Exact Test = 34.021, $p < .001$, Cramér's V = .59), but not for the visual frames (Fisher's Exact Test = .717, p = .68). The results are offered in Table 6.21 and Table 6.22.

Table 6.19 Fisher's Exact Test for Verbal Frames in SIPs and Target Audience

	PLWHA		*African Americans and LGBT*	
Frames	*Count*	*%*	*Count*	*%*
Normal	44	19.0_a	13	28.3_a
Survivor	178	76.7_a	31	67.4_a
Victim	10	4.3_a	1	2.2_a
Carrier	0		1	2.2_b

Note: * $p < .05$ ** $p < .01$ *** $p < .001$. Subscript letters indicate pairs that are significantly different (Bonferroni correction).

Table 6.20 Fisher's Exact Test for Visual Frames in SIPs and Target Audience

	PLWHA		*African Americans and LGBT*	
Frames	*Count*	*%*	*Count*	*%*
Normal	39	84.8_a	9	81.8_a
Survivor	1	2.2_a	1	9.1_a
Victim	4	8.7_a	1	9.1_a
Carrier	2	4.3_a	0	—

Note: * $p < .05$ ** $p < .01$ *** $p < .001$. Subscript letters indicate pairs that are significantly different (Bonferroni correction).

Table 6.21 Fisher's Exact Test for Verbal Frames in PSAs and PSA-Type

	Prevention		*Treatment and Anti-stigma*	
Frames	*Count*	*%*	*Count*	*%*
Normal	58	77.3_a	4	16.0_b^{***}
Survivor	13	17.3_a	19	76.0_b^{***}
Victim	3	4.0_a	0	—
Carrier	1	1.3_a	2	8.0_a

Note: * $p < .05$ ** $p < .01$ *** $p < .001$. Subscript letters indicate pairs that are significantly different (Bonferroni correction).

Table 6.22 Fisher's Exact Test for Visual Frames in PSAs and PSA-Type

	Prevention		*Treatment and Anti-stigma*	
Frames	*Count*	*%*	*Count*	*%*
Normal	54	96.4_a	52	92.9_a
Survivor	2	3.6_a	4	7.1_a

Note: * $p < .05$ ** $p < .01$ *** $p < .001$. Subscript letters indicate pairs that are significantly different (Bonferroni correction).

Table 6.21 shows the result of cross-tabbing verbal frames in PSAs with the variable recording the type of PSA. As shown, statistically significant differences were found in that the normal frame was used significantly more in prevention PSAs (77.3%) than in treatment and anti-stigma PSAs (16.0%). The survivor frame was used significantly more in treatment and anti-stigma PSAs (76.0%) than in prevention PSAs (17.3%). No significant differences were observed for the visual frames (Table 6.22).

Variations by Characteristics of the PLWHA

H5a predicted that the victim and the carrier frames would be used significantly more for PLWHA who are female, homosexual/bisexual, or non-white than for those who are male, heterosexual, or white. In turn, H5b posed that the normal and the survivor frames would be used significantly more for PLWHA who are male, heterosexual, or white than for those who are female, homosexual/bisexual, or non-white.

To test H5a and H5b, a variable recording the verbal frames was crosstabbed with one recording gender (male/female) and one recording sexual orientation (heterosexual vs. bisexual and homosexual)—as this information was collected on the basis of the verbal component of the messages in sample. Also, as information about race/ethnicity was extracted from the visuals, one variable recording the visual frames was crosstabbed with the one recording race/ethnicity[17] (white vs. non-white). As shown in Table 6.23, significant differences in the verbal frames used were noticed by gender (Fisher's Exact Test = 38.168, $p < .001$ [Monte Carlo method], Cramér's V = .267) and sexual orientation (Fisher's Exact Test = 30.201, $p < .005$ [Monte Carlo method], Cramér's V = .334). Also, as seen in Table 6.24, significant differences were found between the use of visual frames by race/ethnicity (Fisher's Exact Test = 25.376, $p < .001$ [Monte Carlo method], Cramér's V = .311). However, these differences were generally not as predicted.

H5a was rejected. While no significant differences were noticed in the use of the victim frame by gender, the carrier frame was employed significantly more for male than for female PLWHA in news (9.7% vs. 1.9%; see Table 6.23). Also in news, the victim frame was used significantly more for white PLWHA (8.1%) than for non-white PLWHA (0.8%) (see Table 6.24). No significant differences by sexual orientation were observed in the way the victim and carrier frames were employed.

Partial support was found for H5b. As predicted, the normal frame was conveyed significantly more for male than for female PLWHA in

Table 6.23 Fisher's Exact Test for Verbal Frames and PLWHA's Gender and Sexual Orientation (Monte Carlo)

		Gender				*Sexual Orientation*			
		Male		*Female*		*Heterosexual*		*Homosexual or Bisexual*	
Context	*Frames*	*Count*	*%*	*Count*	*%*	*Count*	*%*	*Count*	*%*
News	Normal	45	11.8_a	6	3.9_b***	15	11.9_a	25	16.9_a
	Survivor	28	7.3_a	12	7.8_a	16	12.7_a	10	6.8_a
	Victim	19	5.0_a	8	5.2_a	7	5.6_a	6	4.1_a
	Carrier	37	9.7_a	3	1.9_b***	17	13.5_a	13	8.8_a
SIPs	Normal	33	8.6_a	24	15.6_b***	15	11.9_a	21	14.2_a
	Survivor	153	40.1_a	56	36.4_a	21	16.7_a	55	37.2_b***
	Victim	9	2.4_a	2	1.3_a	2	1.6_a	5	3.4_a
	Carrier	1	0.3_a	0	0	1	0.8_a	0	0
PSAs	Normal	34	8.9_a	28	18.2_b***	17	13.5_a	8	5.4_b***
	Survivor	17	4.5_a	15	9.7_b***	10	7.9_a	4	2.7_b***
	Victim	3	0.8_a	0	0	2	1.6_a	1	0.7_a
	Carrier	3	0.8_a	0	0	3	2.4_a	0	0

Note: * $p < .05$ ** $p < .01$ *** $p < .001$. Subscript letters indicate pairs that are significantly different (Bonferroni correction).

Table 6.24 Fisher's Exact Test for Visual Frames and PLWHA's Race/Ethnicity

		Race/Ethnicity			
		White		*Non-white*	
Context	*Frames*	*Count*	%	*Count*	%
News	Normal	27	20.0_a	22	17.5_a
	Survivor	24	17.8_a	7	5.6_b**
	Victim	11	8.1_a	1	0.8_b**
	Carrier	10	7.4_a	10	7.9_a
SIPs	Normal	15	11.1_a	18	14.3_a
	Survivor	1	0.7_a	0	—
	Victim	0	—	3	2.4_a
	Carrier	0	—	0	—
PSAs	Normal	45	33.3_a	61	48.4_b**
	Survivor	2	1.5_a	4	3.2_a
	Victim	0	—	0	—
	Carrier	0	—	0	—

Note: * $p < .05$ ** $p < .01$ *** $p < .001$. Subscript letters indicate pairs that are significantly different (Bonferroni correction).

news (11.8% vs. 3.9%). But contrary to my prediction, the normal frame was used significantly more for female than for male PLWHA in both SIPs (15.6% vs. 8.6%) and PSAs (18.2% vs. 8.9%). The survivor frame was conveyed in PSAs significantly more for female than for male PLWHA (9.7% vs. 4.5%; see Table 6.23).

As for sexual orientation, no significant differences existed in the way the four frames of interest were conveyed in news. As predicted, however, both the normal and the survivor frames were conveyed significantly more for heterosexuals than for bisexual and homosexual PLWHA in PSAs: normal frame (13.5% vs. 5.4%) and survivor frame (7.9% vs. 2.7%). In SIPs, however, the survivor frame was used significantly more for bisexual and homosexual PLWHA than for heterosexual PLWHA (37.2% vs. 16.7%).

Finally, moving to race/ethnicity, the results obtained for the survivor frame confirm the prediction made in H5b, but those for the normal frame contradict it. Specifically, in news, the survivor frame was used significantly more for white PLWHA (17.8%) than for non-white PLWHA (5.6%). However, in PSAs, the normal frame was conveyed significantly more for non-white (48.4%) than for white PLWHA (33.3%).

No other significant paired comparisons existed (see Tables 6.23 and 6.24).

Variations by Nonverbal Behavior and Structural Features

H6 predicted that the nonverbal behavior exhibited by PLWHA depicted through the survivor and normal frames would be significantly more positive than that displayed by PLWHA depicted through the victim or carrier frame. This hypothesis was tested with the help of a two-way ANOVA using the variable recording the overall valence of nonverbal behavior through the Janis Fadner Coefficient of Imbalance (JFCoI, Janis & Fadner, 1949) as a dependent variable and the following two variables as independent variables: communication context (news, SIPs, PSAs) and visual frames (normal, survivor, victim, carrier).

To compute the JFCoI, the following steps were pursued. First, all scores coded "favorable" were added in a new variable called "F"; they were: the PLWHA shown looked directly into the camera; had upturned mouth corners; active hands; arms at shoulder height; stood tall; and was located above other people shown in the same picture. Second, all scores coded "unfavorable" were added in a new variable called "U"; they were the PLWHA shown looked away from the camera; had downturned mouth corners; passive hands; lowered arms; was sitting, lying, or was hunched over; and was depicted beneath other people shown in the same photo. Third, all scores coded "neutral" were added in a new variable called "N"; they were the PLWHA shown was depicted at the same level as others, and her or his mouth corners were relaxed (see Table 3.1). Fourth, seven new variables needed to calculate the "JFCoI" were computed; they were "R" = F + U + N; "F^2"=F * F; "R^2"=R * R; "U^2"=U * U; "FU"=F * U; "CF" (if F > U) = (F^2 – FU)/R^2; "CU" (if F < U) = (FU – U^2)/R^2. Finally, JFCoI was computed by adding the coefficient of favorable imbalance "CF" and the coefficient of unfavorable imbalance "CU"; values could, in principle, range from +1.0 to –1.0.

In this way, the JFCoI did not just add up differently valenced nonverbal behavior cues but rather took into account the difference in the proportions of positive, negative, and balanced/neutral nonverbal behavior for each PLWHA in sample. It eliminated the problem of positive and negative values annulling each other when the various variables were summed. The JFCoI increased whenever the frequency of positive nonverbal behavior increased and decreased whenever the frequency of negative nonverbal behavior increased. The value was set at zero when just as many indicators of positive and negative nonverbal behavior were encountered, and when the nonverbal information was neutral.

Frequencies, means, and standard deviations for the JFCoI are offered in Table 6.25. No significant differences in the valence of nonverbal behavior were noticed due to either communication context $F(2, 252) = .94$, $p = .39$, visual frame $F(3, 252) = .09$, $p = .97$, or the interaction between these two independent variables $F(3, 252) = .99$, $p = .40$. H6 was rejected.

H7 tested whether there were significant differences in the use of camera angles among the four visual frames. The procedure involved the use of crosstabs between a variable recording the visual frames (normal, survivor, victim, carrier) and a variable recording camera angles (high, eye-level, low). H7a predicted that the normal, victim, and carrier frames would use significantly more eye-level camera angles than would the survivor frames. H7b posed that survivor frames would use significantly more low-level camera angles than would the normal, victim, and carrier frames. H7c anticipated that victim frames would use significantly more high-level camera angles than would the normal, victim, and carrier frames. These hypotheses were tested using Fisher's Exact Test and rejected (Fisher's Exact Test = 9.817, $p = .07$). The results are offered in Table 6.26.

H8a posed that the normal and survivor frames would use significantly more medium and long shots than would the victim and carrier frames. H8b predicted that victim and carrier frames would use significantly

Table 6.25 Frequencies, Means, and Standard Deviations for the Janis–Fadner Coefficient of Imbalance per Visual Frame

		Valence of Nonverbal Behavior		
Context	*Frame*	*n*	*M*	*SD*
News	Normal	49	−0.01	0.33
	Survivor	31	0.19	0.24
	Victim	12	−0.02	0.39
	Carrier	20	0.04	0.39
SIPs	Normal	33	0.02	0.31
	Victim	3	0.04	0.25
	Survivor	1	0.00	—
PSAs	Normal	106	0.19	0.27
	Survivor	6	0.16	0.27

Table 6.26 Fisher's Exact Test for Visual Frames and Camera Angles

	Frames							
	Normal		*Survivor*		*Victim*		*Carrier*	
	Count	%	*Count*	%	*Count*	%	*Count*	%
High	3	1.5_a	2	4.9_a	1	5.9_a	0	—
Eye-level	197	96.1_a	35	85.4_b	15	$88.2_{a,b}$	22	$100.0_{a,b}$
Low	5	2.4_a	4	9.8_a	1	5.9_a	0	—

Note: * $p < .05$ ** $p < .01$ *** $p < .001$. Subscript letters indicate pairs that are significantly different.

more close-ups than would normal and survivor frames. The procedure was a crosstab between a variable recording the visual frames (normal, survivor, victim, carrier) and one recording camera distances (close-ups, medium shots, long shots). The Fisher's Exact Test provided some support for these hypotheses: Fisher's Exact Test = 86.564, $p < .001$, Cramér's V = .507. Results are offered in Table 6.27.

As predicted by H8a, long shots were used significantly more for the normal (45.4%) and survivor frames (70.7%) than for the carrier frame (13.6%). No significant differences between the normal and survivor frames on the one hand and the victim frame on the other were observed. Medium shots were used significantly more when a normal frame was conveyed (50.2%) than when a carrier frame was conveyed (13.6%). No other significant paired comparisons existed (see Table 6.27).

H8b was partly supported. As seen in Table 6.27, the carrier frame used significantly more close-ups (81.8%) than the normal frame and the victim frames (4.4% and 11.8%, respectively) did. Contrary to my prediction, no significant differences between the victim frame and the normal and survivor frames were found with regard to the use of close-ups.

Also, given that three different communication contexts are analyzed in this study, it seemed worthwhile to investigate whether the above reported differences might also be rooted in the communication context, not just in the visual frames. A Fisher's Exact Test was conducted to test this possibility and found significant differences, Fisher's Exact Test (Monte Carlo) = 123.250, $p < .001$, Cramér's V = .326. As shown in Table 6.28, significantly more close-ups were used in SIPs (52.2%) than in news (20.6%) and PSAs (7.5%). On the other hand, significantly more medium shots were used in PSAs (63.7%) than in news (33.8%) and SIPs (28.3%). Finally, significantly more long shots were employed in news (45.6%) than in PSAs (28.8%) and SIPs (19.6%).

Table 6.27 Fisher's Exact Test for Visual Frames and Camera Distances

	Frames							
	Normal		*Survivor*		*Victim*		*Carrier*	
	Count	*%*	*Count*	*%*	*Count*	*%*	*Count*	*%*
Close-up	9	4.4_{a}	0		2	11.8_{a}	18	81.8_{b}
Medium shot	103	50.2_{a}***	12	$29.3_{a,\ b}$	4	$23.5_{a,\ b}$	1	4.5_{b}***
Long shot	93	45.4_{a}***	29	70.7_{b}***	11	$64.7_{a,\ b}$	3	13.6_{c}***

Note: * $p < .05$ ** $p < .01$ *** $p < .001$. Subscript letters indicate pairs that are significantly different (Bonferroni correction).

Verbal-Visual Frame Congruence

In this section, the last research question and the last two hypotheses are addressed. They dealt with the relationship between verbal frames and visual frames. Investigating the way verbal frames relate to visual frames meant carrying out the last step in the integrative framing analysis (see Figure 5.1).

A one-way ANOVA between a variable measuring the verbal-visual frame congruence ratio[18] (interval, values between –1.0 and +1.0) and a variable recording communication context (news, SIPs, PSA) was used to test H9. This hypothesis posed that the verbal-visual frame congruence ratio would be higher for PSAs than for SIPs and news. The analysis found support for this hypothesis, Welch's F (2, 182) = 8.791, $p < .001$, $\eta^2 = .09$. Dunnett C post-hoc tests revealed that the congruence ratio in PSAs ($M = .74$, $SD = .44$, $n = 76$) was significantly higher than in news ($M = .44$, $SD = .49$, $n = 70$) and SIPs ($M = .45$, $SD = .50$, $n = 39$), respectively (see Table 6.29).

Table 6.28 Fisher's Exact Test for Communication Contexts and Camera Distances (Monte Carlo)

	Context					
	News		*SIPs*		*PSAs*	
	Count	*%*	*Count*	*%*	*Count*	*%*
Close-up	42	20.6_a^{***}	120	52.2_b^{***}	11	7.5_c^{***}
Medium shot	69	33.8_a	65	28.3_a	93	63.7_b^{***}
Long shot	93	45.6_a^{***}	45	19.6_b	42	28.8_b

Note: * $p < .05$ ** $p < .01$ *** $p < .001$. Subscript letters indicate pairs that are significantly different (Bonferroni correction).

Table 6.29 Multiple Comparisons (Dunnett C) between the Communication Contexts on the Dependent Variable Congruence Ratio

(I) Communication Context	*(J) Communication Context*	*Mean Difference (I – J)*	*Standard Error*	*95% Confidence Interval*	
				Lower Bound	*Upper Bound*
News	SIPs	–0.01	0.09	–0.24	0.23
	PSAs	$-.29^{***}$	0.08	–0.49	–0.10
SIPs	News	0.01	0.09	–0.23	0.24
	PSAs	$-.28^{**}$	0.09	–0.52	–0.06
PSAs	News	$.29^{***}$	0.08	0.10	0.49
	SIPs	$.28^{**}$	0.09	0.06	0.52

Note: * $p < .05$ ** $p < .01$ *** $p < .001$.

RQ2 asked whether there were any statistically significant differences in the congruence ratio based on (1) the characteristics of the state in which the newspaper was published, (2) the target audience of the SIPs, or (3) the PSA type.

A three-way ANOVA was computed between the congruence ratio and the following characteristics of the state in which the newspaper was published: conservatism, urbanism, religiosity, and HIV/AIDS prevalence. There was no statistically significant interaction between the congruence ratio and any of the following: conservatism $F(1, 63) = 1.456$, $p = .232$, observed power = .221; religiosity $F(1, 63) = .021$, $p = .884$, observed power = .052; HIV/AIDS prevalence $F(1, 63) = 2.676$, $p = .107$, observed power = .364; urbanism $F(1, 63) = 3.330$, $p = .073$, observed power = .435. There was no significant three-way interaction. Frequencies, means, and standard deviations are offered in Table 6.30.

Next, a one-way ANOVA was used to investigate whether the congruence ratio between verbal frames and visual frames in SIPs varied significantly by target audience (PLWHA vs. African Americans and LGBT). This was not the case, Welch's $F(1, 37) = .309$, $p = .59$ (see Table 6.31).

Finally, a one-way ANOVA was calculated between the congruence ratio between verbal frames and visual frames in PSAs, and the PSA type. Significant differences were observed, Welch's $F(1, 74) = 27.47$, $p < .001$, $\eta^2 = .35$ (see Table 6.32). Specifically, the congruence ratio was

Table 6.30 Frequencies, Means, and Standard Deviations for the State Characteristic per Congruence Ratio

		Congruence Ratio		
		n	*M*	*SD*
State Characteristics				
Conservatism				
	Low	42	.53	.10
	High	28	.31	.12
Urbanism				
	Low	13	.21	.15
	High	57	.61	.08
Religiosity				
	Low	41	.41	.11
	High	29	.48	.11
HIV/AIDS Prevalence				
	Low	49	.28	.09
	High	21	.85	.14

Table 6.31 Welch's *F*-Test of Verbal-Visual Frame Congruence Ratio in SIPs for Target Audience

	Congruence Ratio		
	n	*M*	*SD*
Target Audience			
PLWHA	32	.47	.51
African Americans and LGBT	7	.36	.48

Note: * $p < .05$ ** $p < .01$ *** $p < .001$.

Table 6.32 Welch's F-Test of Verbal-Visual Frame Congruence Ratio in PSAs for PSA Type

	Congruence Ratio			
	n	*M*	*SD*	η^2
PSA Type				
Prevention	56	.89***	.31	.35
Treatment and anti-stigma	20	.30***	.47	.35

Note: * $p < .05$ ** $p < .01$ *** $p < .001$.

significantly higher for prevention PSAs ($M = .89$, $SD = .31$, $n = 56$) than for treatment and anti-stigma PSAs ($M = .30$, $SD = .47$, $n = 20$).

H10 posed that the verbal-visual frame congruence ratio would vary significantly according to the verbal frame conveyed. In other words, it was posed that the verbal frame conveyed would have an effect on the likelihood that this frame would be matched by its visual expression in the accompanying photo(s).

This hypothesis was tested using a one-way ANOVA between the congruence ratio and a variable recording the verbal frame. As predicted, the verbal frame had a significant effect on the congruence ratio, $F(3, 181) = 37.286$, $p < .001$, $\eta^2 = .38$. The results of the Tukey HSD post-hoc test are offered in Table 6.33.

The congruence ratio was significantly higher when a normal frame was conveyed ($M = .83$, $SD = .38$, $n = 87$) than when a survivor ($M = .17$, $SD = .37$, $n = 56$) or a victim frame were used ($M = .27$, $SD = .43$, $n = 18$). Also, the congruence ratio was significantly higher when the verbal frame conveyed was carrier ($M = .75$, $SD = .44$, $n = 24$) as opposed to both the survivor ($M = .17$, $SD = .37$, $n = 56$) and the victim frames ($M = .27$, $SD = .43$, $n = 18$).

Table 6.33 Multiple Comparisons (Tukey HSD) between the Verbal Frames on the Dependent Variable Congruence Ratio

(I) Verbal Frame	*(J) Verbal Frame*	*Mean Difference (I – J)*	*Standard Error*	*95% Confidence Interval*	
				Lower Bound	*Upper Bound*
Normal	Survivor	.66***	.07	.48	.83
	Victim	.55***	.10	.29	.81
	Carrier	.08	.09	–.16	.31
Survivor	Normal	–.66***	.07	–.83	–.48
	Victim	–.11	.11	–.38	.17
	Carrier	–.58***	.10	–.83	–.33
Victim	Normal	–.55***	.10	–.81	–.29
	Survivor	.11	.11	–.17	.38
	Carrier	–.47**	.12	–.79	–.16
Carrier	Normal	–.08	.09	–.31	.16
	Survivor	.58***	.10	.33	.83
	Victim	.47**	.12	.16	.79

Note: * $p < .05$ ** $p < .01$ *** $p < .001$. Subscript letters indicate pairs that are significantly different (Bonferroni correction).

Discussion

The empirical analysis presented above was conducted to demonstrate the approach to integrative framing analysis developed in Chapter 5. The focus was placed on the verbal and visual frames conveyed for PLWHA in various communication contexts. Such frames about people are known in the literature as character frames (Grabe & Bucy, 2009). Investigating character frames is worthwhile, as they inform about how journalists and other actors communicate about people most directly affected by an issue. This, in turn, can affect the way audiences think of the issue as a whole more than baseline statistics (Sharf & Vandeford, 2003). For instance, the framing of refugees and asylum seekers may play an important role in the way audiences think and feel about the issue of migration, just as the framing of people out of work can affect beliefs about the issue of unemployment.

This study found that all four frames of interest (normal, survivor, victim, carrier) were encountered in the verbal component of news, SIPs, and PSAs. The visual component of news conveyed all four frames, whereas three of the four frames were conveyed in SIPs and only two in PSAs. This finding makes sense considering the various roles journalists on the one hand and advocates on the other play in society. From a normative perspective, journalists are expected to be objective and to present as many sides of the story as are relevant and ultimately serve the public good (Baerns, 1991). Advocates, on the other hand, may advance just their side of the story in the hope that it will help reach their individual interests, which may or may not align with the public interest (Baerns, 1991; Hänggli & Kriesi, 2012; Van Gorp, 2010). These results suggest that journalists do, indeed, try to present more sides of the story than advocates do. Similar findings were obtained in previous research, where various advocate materials conveyed just one or two frames per issue (Gilman, 1995; Grover, 1992), whereas news frames were much more diversified (Crimp, 1992; Lupton, 1999).

Another interpretation could be that the visual repertoire of journalists was more sophisticated than that of SIPs contributors and public health officials. But it may be wrong to assume that public health officials, especially, were unable to convey all four frames visually. These officials have sufficient means to pretest their messages; they could also outsource this task should they lack expertise. It may be that public health officials choose to refrain from visual carrier and victim frames. Not having surveyed or interviewed SIPs contributors and public health officials, I cannot shed light on the reasons behind these framing decisions. Future research could address this.

In response to H1a, this study found that the victim and carrier frames were used significantly more in the verbal component of news than in that of SIPs and PSAs. Also, in response to H1b, the normal frame was more common in PSA texts than in news texts, whereas the survivor frame was used more in SIPs texts than in news texts. Moreover, while no significant differences among the communication contexts were noticed with regard to the visual expression of the victim and carrier frames, the visual normal frame was much more common in SIPs and PSAs (about 90% each) than in news (about 40%). The visual survivor frame was more common in news (about 20%) than in both SIPs and PSAs (on average 4% each). As already suggested above, these results are likely the product of journalists' striving for balance and advocates' attempting to promote their preferred frames.

From the perspective of journalism and communication studies, these results are encouraging. They suggest that journalists are, indeed, trying to present as many sides of the story as possible (Baerns, 1991), despite the fact that the frame advocates included in this study might want them to act differently. However, since journalists use not just the positive frames preferred by advocates (normal, survivor), but also the negative ones (victim, carrier), a more nuanced discussion seems in order. Specifically, is the journalistic use of the victim and carrier frames legitimate?

These frames can perpetuate stigma and stereotypes and hurt the feelings of those directly affected. News stories doing this do not stand good chances to contribute to community building and some scholars might criticize this (Franklin & Parry, 1998; Kaniss, 1991). Also, the victim and carrier frames may not be conducive to public health (Aggleton & Parker, 2002; Alonzo & Reynolds, 1995). Indeed, some see journalists as responsible for the health of their readers (e.g., DeSilva, Muskavitch, & Roche, 2004; Mebane, Temin, & Parvanta, 2003; Swain, 2007). While I am sympathetic to this line of reasoning, I believe it is public health officials who are responsible for the health of the population, not journalists. Thus, I would argue that journalists cannot be expected to act as proxies for the efforts of activists and public health officials. In any case, surveys and interviews with health journalists suggested that many of them reject the implicit expectation that they should "put aside investigation reporting skills" (Whitaker, 2013, p. 147) just because the matters they cover are immediately relevant to people's lives (see also Donohue, Tichenor, & Olien, 1995; Evensen & Clarke, 2012). As welcome as it may be that news sometimes contributes to bringing the members of a community together (as opposed to dividing them), this appears nowhere near the job description of journalists. Demanding that journalists only report in a positive manner is out of place, especially when they would have to hold back legitimate information to do this.

The carrier and victim frames convey a more blunt/accurate picture of the issue of HIV/AIDS than the frames preferred by advocates (normal and survivor). Experimental research suggested that presenting those affected by a medical condition in too positive a light may be met with skepticism anyway (Niederdeppe, Shapiro, & Roh, 2014). Showing both the good and the bad aspects of issues can increase trust in the information presented. It appears that some PLWHA actually behave in ways that justify the use of victim and carrier frames. Thus, the goal cannot be for journalists to self-censor in such a way to make these frames disappear from coverage. However, these frames may be overrepresented; this possibility is discussed below in the context of the findings for H2.

I now move to the discussion of the small number of frames and their nature in SIPs and PSAs. They, too, were obtained in response to H1a and H1b. These hypotheses were partly supported. One finding was that the victim and the carrier frames were used in less than 5% of the SIPs texts and in less than 10% of the SIPs photos. As the SIPs in sample target audiences which, according to the CDC (2015a), are most affected by HIV/AIDS, it makes sense that SIPs contributors seemed to prefer normal and survivor frames. Unlike journalists, SIPs contributors cannot be expected to be balanced or objective. It is neither their function nor their goal. From this perspective, I do not consider the finding worrisome that SIPs may indeed use the frames that their audiences are likely to prefer. However, there is a possibility that these publications' confinement to the positive frames may have a negative impact on social cohesion. This is something addressed below in more depth in the discussion of the results obtained for H3.

The finding that only 6% of the PSAs analyzed in this study verbally conveyed victim and carrier frames and that none of them conveyed these frames visually is surprising. Indeed, previous studies reported tendencies to the contrary in the early days of the epidemic (Hallet & Cannella, 1994; Hammond, 1997). It may be that public health officials rejected victim and carrier frames as not conducive to public health. This explanation seems plausible when one considers previous research findings on how the perpetuation of stigma goes hand-in-hand with the perpetuation of the epidemic (Aggleton & Parker, 2002; Alonzo & Reynolds, 1995). However, this also could be the result of having sampled only materials in which PLWHA were shown or referenced. This criterion allowed the selection of a relevant and manageable sample, but it also meant that CDC's prevention PSAs were not included in the analysis. Thus, it is not clear whether the result that PSAs use predominantly normal and survivor frames would also hold true for prevention PSAs by the CDC. Future framing analyses of CDC's prevention PSAs could settle this matter.

It is also important to note that an evaluation of carrier and victim frames from a public health perspective would be best if informed by experimental research into the effects of the four frames on audiences. This has not been the focus of the present study, but it constitutes a way in which this study could be continued. Scholars could investigate framing effects on attitudes, behavior and behavioral intentions toward PLWHA, willingness to engage in prevention behavior, cognition, or emotion (see Dan & Coleman, 2014).

This study posed that there would be a connection between verbal frames and news sources on the one hand and visual frames and photo sources on the other (H2a, H2b). This was deemed important, because news frames are likely to be shaped at least in part by sources providing information and visuals. These hypotheses were supported. Analogous to previous research, the news frames differed significantly among the news sources used (e.g., Dimitrova & Strömbäck, 2012; Strömbäck et al., 2013). Also, significant differences in the visual frames were observed among photo sources. To my knowledge, this study is the first to show the connection between sources and visual frames.

The analysis revealed that the normal and survivor frames were predominant when nonprofit organizations and PLWHA, their friends, or family were used as news sources. Also, the normal frame was conveyed in news stories where medical institutions acted as news sources. These results are not surprising. Indeed, it makes sense that these frames are preferred by these news sources. No significant differences were observed for the victim frame.

Perhaps the most interesting finding here was that the carrier frame was conveyed more, both verbally and visually, when news sources from law enforcement institutions were used than any other news sources.

This suggests that law enforcement institutions may help journalists achieve their goal of a balanced coverage of HIV/AIDS. Law enforcement institutions are perhaps among the few who can also tell this part of the story to journalists—namely that, unfortunately, some PLWHA do spread the virus intentionally. Previous research suggested that audiences are interested in crime news (Ericson, Baranek, & Chan, 1989; O'Neill & O'Connor, 2008; Trautman, 2004). Scholars also discussed the importance of crime news for public safety and welfare, making it a duty for journalists to report on this (Potter & Kappeler, 1998).

It is possible that activists and public health officials would like to sensitize journalists and law enforcement institutions to the potentially detrimental effects of the carrier frame or even to try to make the carrier frame disappear from the news. It is unlikely that they would succeed, however, given that, as long as some PLWHA spread the virus intentionally, journalists striving to be objective are unlikely to refrain from using the carrier frame. Perhaps public health officers, NGOs, activists, and journalists could work together to establish a common understanding of what balanced coverage means. For instance, advocates could try to determine how many of the PLWHA feel and act in ways synonymous to the normal, survivor, victim, and carrier frame, respectively. Advocates could provide this information to journalists. It would then be up to journalists to try to reproduce these circumstances in their coverage—as difficult as that may be. If only 1% of the PLWHA spread the virus intentionally, then this would mean that these individuals are overrepresented in the media coverage and that stigma and discrimination could proliferate as a result.

I believe the results reported above attest to the importance of investigating the way verbal and visual news frames vary among the news sources and photo sources used (frame building). I hope that future studies will consider continuing the investigation of differences in framing not just among news sources but also among photo sources. For the verbal part of the analysis, researchers might want to record news sources not for the entire news article, as done in this study, but for each sentence in the news article individually. This would allow a more in-depth evaluation of news sources' contribution to news framing.

In this study, much effort was put into the selection of a sample as diverse as possible. News texts and news photos originating in 24 news outlets were analyzed; they were published in states that varied in prevailing political views, religious views, degree of urbanism, and the prevalence of HIV/AIDS. This seemed important, as previous research suggested that attitudes toward PLWHA varied by these characteristics. Moreover, articles from five special-interest publications were analyzed. These SIPs were directed at PLWHA, African Americans, and members of the LGBT community, respectively. Finally, unlike many existing studies, this one examined not just prevention PSAs, but also

PSAs focused on things beside prevention (i.e., PSAs advocating against stigma and discrimination and PSAs urging PLWHA to start/continue treatment). Several hypotheses and research questions investigated how, if at all, these variations were consequential for the framing of PLWHA.

One finding was that the news framing differed significantly according to several state characteristics. H3 was partly supported. Specifically, the positive frames (normal and survivor) were more frequent in the verbal news coverage from states with high HIV/AIDS rates, high urbanism, low conservatism, and low religiosity than in news from states with the opposite characteristics. Similarly, the verbal expression of the victim frame was more typical of news from states characterized by low conservatism and low religiosity than in conservative and religious states. Conversely, the carrier frame was more prevalent in news from states with high conservatism, high religiosity, low HIV/AIDS rates, and low urbanism.

Support for these results appears in previous studies using public opinion surveys, focus groups, and experiments (e.g., Dhooper & Royse, 1989; Doka, 1997; Mondragón et al., 1991; Muturi & An, 2010; Patterson, 2014). I find it interesting that my results, which were obtained through content analysis, go hand-in-hand with those obtained by others using human subjects. This increases my confidence in the finding that people's thoughts and feelings toward PLWHA are a function of their residence, the prevalence of HIV/AIDS in the region, and of their political and religious views.

These results can be interpreted in several ways. First, it may be that journalists, as residents of a certain state, hold the same views as the majority of the population in that state. From this perspective, it makes sense that journalists in states with different characteristics would cover PLWHA differently. But previous research generally suggests that journalists' individual characteristics are among the least powerful factors influencing news coverage (see Shoemaker & Reese, 2014). It may be that HIV/AIDS is one of the issues in which journalists' personal views surface in the coverage. An alternative explanation would be that local journalists, in an attempt to act as "good neighbors" (Poindexter et al., 2006), covered HIV/AIDS in a way that fully acknowledged how their respective communities were made up. Such influences were described in a large number of studies conducted through the community structure approach (Pollock, 2007). However, the findings in framing scholarship were mixed (Liebler & Bendix, 1996; McLemore, 2015). Future research involving surveys or interviews with health journalists could help shed more light on which of these two interpretations is more plausible.

Another explanation could be that news frames are not necessarily frames preferred by journalists but rather the frames constructed in interaction with news sources, even though journalists may use news sources deliberately (Hagen, 1993). It is possible that the differences

I noticed in news framing were due not to the way prevailing values and views in the state affected journalists, but rather to how these values and views affected local frame advocates acting as news sources. This would mean that the characteristics of the state influenced news coverage indirectly, by influencing news sources. Future research could try to demonstrate this hypothesis of vicarious influence.

From a practical perspective, the result that predominant views are reproduced and legitimized in news highlights once again the importance of designing public communication campaigns geared to the target group. Indeed, one-message-fits-all national campaigns promoting, say, the equal treatment of PLWHA, might be ineffective in rural, very religious, very conservative communities with low HIV/AIDS prevalence where the media coverage uses the carrier frame. Local campaigns with customized messages might be more effective. When designing messages for more conservative audiences, public health communicators might do the opposite of what they normally do. Specifically, instead of conveying just the one or two frames they prefer, they could also acknowledge competing frames and justify why they reject them. It is possible that such balanced messages can help convey that while certain unflattering stereotypes may be applicable to some PLWHA, they are not the only way in which one can think of PLWHA. There is a fairly good chance that such local campaigns exist, but they were not included in this study. Future research could, perhaps, pair local news coverage with local advocate frames. To identify local advocates, scholars could first investigate the news sources used by local journalists before sampling advocacy materials.

On a more philosophical note, the result that people's religious and political views got reproduced in the media coverage of PLWHA is worrisome, because it might mean that people get exposed predominantly to news frames compatible to their own worldviews (see Bryant & Davies, 2008). This could widen the rift between the proponents of conflicting views and, in the long run, jeopardize social cohesion (see Gandy, 2001).

As for the visual frames, the only significant difference based on state characteristics was that the carrier frame was conveyed more in news from states with low HIV/AIDS rates than in their counterparts. The explanations provided above in response to variations in verbal news framing might also apply here. It may also be that journalists in states where HIV/AIDS rates are high refrain from reproducing police mug shots in stories about PLWHA accused of crimes, if not from covering these stories altogether. For instance, several articles in my sample reported that a priest living with HIV/AIDS had been accused of indecent exposure and sex solicitation. Some news articles used photos of this priest in the court of law surrounded by lawyers, law enforcement officers, and so on. Yet, despite the apparent availability of such carrier-framed photos, other journalists/media ran favorable stock photos instead. They showed the man performing worship services in a church (Shaffer, 2013). Previous literature suggested that when words convey meanings different from those conveyed visually, people will remember the visual interpretation of the issue (Kobayashi, 1986; Paivio & Csapo, 1973). Thus, choosing a favorable stock photo to accompany a news article describing the priest's alleged actions in depth can be seen as downplaying those accusations. If journalists aim for balance, it would be best to convey the same meaning in words and visuals. In case journalists want to portray the accused as untypical—and a typical mug shot was deemed as unable to convey this message—then a juxtaposition between a stock photo and a mug shot might be the answer.

In this study, the target audience of the SIPs did not have a significant impact on the frames used in these publications. It seemed reasonable to assume that SIPs targeted at PLWHA would convey different frames from those targeted at LGBT and African Americans (H4). That this was not the case may be due to these target audiences not being dissimilar enough. Future research could draw a more diverse sample of SIPs. For instance, in light of the results discussed in the above paragraph, SIPs that target religious or conservative audiences—the *Christian Post,* for instance—could be included in the analysis. There is a good chance that the frames used in, say *POZ* magazine—which is directed at PLWHA—are different from those used in the *Christian Post.*

The last finding concerning the impact of the medium characteristics on the framing of PLWHA concerns the influence of the PSA type (RQ1). This study found that prevention PSAs conveyed predominantly the normal frame, whereas PSAs advocating against stigma and discrimination and PSAs advocating treatment used the survivor frame most. These differences were only observed in the verbal frames. No significant differences among the different types of PSAs existed in the visual frames.

Public health officials may have resorted to the normal frame in prevention PSAs to communicate that anyone could contract HIV. Ideally, such messages would lead to an increased identification with the PLWHA featured in the PSA and an elevated awareness of one's own risk.

The finding that public health officials mostly used survivor frames in treatment PSAs may have had to do with motivation. Perhaps they thought that PLWHA refusing treatment or not adhering to it would react to the hyperbolic prospects suggested by the survivor frame—excellent health and internal state—by changing their behavior as desired. Such a strategy could backfire, given the numerous and occasionally very serious side effects of antiretroviral treatment.

Finally, the predominance of the survivor frame in anti-stigma and discrimination PSAs may be the result of an attempt to advocate for others' acceptance of PLWHA.

Future research could inform whether or not the differential conveyance of normal and survivor frames in different types of PSAs resulted from deliberate decisions by public health officials. Indeed, while this explanation seems plausible, drawing conclusions on communication strategies from content analytical data would be premature. In-depth interviews or surveys are needed.

Since the emergence of HIV/AIDS, public opinion about PLWHA has been contingent upon the characteristics of the individuals in question. Many studies suggested that women, bisexual/homosexual individuals, and ethnic/racial minorities have been condemned more than their counterparts. According to previous research, double standards were also applied in communication about PLWHA (Clarke, 1992; Crimp, 1992; de Souza, 2007; DeJong et al., 2001; Gilman, 1995; Kitzinger, 1993, 1995; Sacks, 1996; Treichler, 1999; Watney, 1990a; Wellings, 1988).

The results obtained in response to H5a do not corroborate these authors' findings. No significant differences in the predicted direction were found. Instead, the victim frame was conveyed more for white than non-white PLWHA. Also, the carrier frame was conveyed more for men, not for women. These findings are very surprising. Three explanations are conceivable.

First, things may have changed since the studies on whose basis the hypothesis was formulated were published. The newest one was published almost a decade ago (see above). The possibility that these studies are no longer up-to-date is also suggested by more recent research finding barely any evidence for the stigmatization of racial/ethnic minorities (Coleman & Hatley Major, 2014) or of bisexual/homosexual PLWHA (Dan & Coleman, 2014).

Second, there is a possibility that—despite first impressions—my findings and those obtained in earlier studies do not contradict each other. It may be, for example, that women and minorities were presented in stereotypical ways other than through the victim and the carrier frame—the present study was not designed to capture these alternative stereotypical ways. For instance, women could have been presented as subservient to their partners but, at the same time, through the normal frame. To clarify this, future studies could also record the existence of stigmatizing content not just within but also beyond the frames of interest.

Third, these findings may simply be a result of error in measurement. A source of error could be sampling, as only materials that featured individuals explicitly identified as living with HIV/AIDS were included in the analysis. As already mentioned, this decision was reached in an attempt to draw a relevant sample and keep the project manageable. In principle, it is conceivable that materials excluded from the sample using this criterion were more stigmatizing to women, bisexual/homosexual individuals, and racial/ethnic minorities. For instance, a news article on HIV/AIDS statistics illustrated with a photo of a commercial sex worker (see Treichler, 1999)—whose individual HIV status was not addressed in the accompanying text—would have not been included in the sample.

However, I can state to the best of my knowledge that I had not encountered such stigmatizing content in the news articles, the PSAs, or the SIPs contributions considered for inclusion in this sample.

Significant differences based on the characteristics of the PLWHA were also noticed with regard to the use of the survivor and the normal frames (H5b). These findings are mixed, however, and their interpretation is difficult. Specifically, in news, the normal frame was used more for males than for females. The opposite was found in PSAs and SIPs; the normal frame was used more for females than for males. The survivor frame was used more for female than male PLWHA in PSAs. Results on the differences in framing by the sexual orientation of PLWHA were also mixed. In SIPs, more survivor frames were conveyed for bisexual/homosexual PLWHA than for heterosexuals. In PSAs, the normal and survivor frames were employed more for heterosexual than for bisexual and homosexual PLWHA. As for race/ethnicity, the survivor frame was conveyed more for whites in news, and the normal frame was used more for whites in PSAs.

Taken together, these results do not qualify as convincing evidence that PLWHA who are women, bisexual/homosexual, or non-white are treated more negatively than their counterparts. The differences may rather be the result of pre-testing PSA messages (e.g., perhaps certain frames resonate better with certain subpopulations) or of protagonists' reticence to volunteer information about their sexuality when featured in news, SIPs, or PSAs. The results may have also been skewed by the overrepresentation of bisexual and homosexual individuals in the SIPs sample (two of the publications targeted LGBT). Another explanation could be that the creators of these messages, aware of the criticism of stereotyping minorities, were putting so much effort into preventing this that they ended up stereotyping nonminorities.

In response to H6, I found that there were no significant differences in the valence of nonverbal behavior exhibited by PLWHA among the frames. This is a surprising finding, as the weight of evidence suggested otherwise (e.g., Coleman & Wu, 2015; Grabe & Bucy, 2009). One possible explanation is that most studies finding such differences investigated moving images, while this study analyzed still images. Perhaps nonverbal behavior plays a different role in visual framing based on the type of images used (still vs. moving). Another explanation could be that nonverbal behavior was part of the visual frames, but that the methodology used in this study was not suitable to capture this subtlety. Future studies should re-evaluate whether hypotheses regarding specific behaviors (e.g., gestures, mimics) as opposed to just at valence (JFCoI) are plausible.

When designing this study, it seemed reasonable to assume, for example, that a person's nonverbal behavior would be more positive when that person engaged in some pleasurable activity together with loved ones (normal frame) than, say, in a hospital surrounded by medical personnel and equipment (victim frame). That this was not found in this study suggests that character frames may not rely that much on changes in nonverbal behavior. Perhaps character frames were conveyed mostly through photo content and structural features, for instance through the props and activity shown or through variations in camera distance (see below). It is also conceivable that alterations in the nonverbal behavior of a person shown in a photo are sufficient to change the frame evoked in viewers' minds. However, as previous visual communication research on PLWHA did not suggest that this was the case, visual frames were not operationalized in this study as consisting of nonverbal behavior alone. It is up to future research to establish via experiments whether different visual frames can be conveyed just by changes in the nonverbal behavior of the protagonist. In other words, when everything else remains the same (setting, attire, props, activity, structural features, etc.), do audiences pick up different frames—or the same frame at different intensity—just because the protagonist's nonverbal behavior changed?

In this study, no significant differences were noticed regarding the use of camera angles to convey the frames investigated (H7a–c). Indeed, there was too little variation in the data, in the sense that most photos used eye-level angles. This could suggest that camera people may try to be neutral or may frame their subjects using other means than camera angle variations. Scholars may choose to focus on these other means, should future studies also fail to find differences in this regard.

The findings of this study concerning camera distance serve to reinforce visual communication scholars' call to pay attention to such variations (H8). Long and medium shots were more typical of the normal and survivor frame, whereas close-ups were typically used with the carrier frame. I believe these results suggest that the connotations typically assigned to camera distance settings by political communication researchers (see Coleman, 2010; Grabe & Bucy, 2009) may not be universal. Previous literature often evaluates close-ups positively by saying that they bring the person portrayed closer to the viewer. But I would argue that they also isolate the subject from the environment, which may not be a good thing for PLWHA, as opposed to politicians, for example. Surveys and experiments are needed to test this assumption.

The last findings to be discussed concern the relationship between the verbal frame conveyed for every PLWHA in the sample and the corresponding visual frame/s. Previous research strongly suggested that messages conveying the same meaning in both words and in visuals are more likely to be remembered and recalled accurately than those in which these two channels of communication convey conflicting messages (see Chapter 2). Determining the extent to which the same frame is conveyed both verbally and visually was therefore deemed worthwhile. I developed a formula that allowed me to calculate a verbal-visual frame congruence ratio. I tested whether this ratio varied significantly according to the communication context, the medium characteristics, and the verbal frame conveyed.

In response to H9, I found that the congruence ratio was significantly higher in PSAs than in SIPs and news. Moreover, the ratio was significantly higher for prevention PSAs than for treatment and anti-stigma PSAs. To understand these findings, one must consider the perspective of the communicator—the journalist, the SIPs contributor, and the public health official.

Through PSAs, public health officials attempt to change the attitudes and even behavior of the audience (Faden & Faden, 1978). It makes sense that these communicators pay attention to frame congruence, especially in prevention PSAs, which are their core business (RQ2). After all, according to the literature reviewed in Chapter 2, they stand better chances of achieving this goal when they put across the same message verbally and visually. This finding suggests that these communicators used frame congruence strategically. It is possible that many more actors pay attention to this, in issues other than those that are health related. For instance, it is conceivable that this already happens in the framing of asylum seekers by rightwing politicians; in that of the European Union by Brexit supporters; or in the framing of investment banks by leftwing politicians criticizing capitalism. Future studies can address topics such as these, and are advised to focus not just on news, but also on materials from various advocates in the issue at hand.

The result that the congruence ratio was highest in PSAs is at odds with previous studies finding that the verbal component of PSAs differed from the visual component (e.g., Cappella, Leader, Kang, & White, 2007; Coleman & Hatley Major, 2014). This difference may be due to my investigation of character frames; perhaps the congruence ratio is higher when people directly affected are shown and described. This result could also be typical of PSAs dealing with HIV/AIDS. Coleman and Hatley Major (2014), for instance, investigated PSAs on several health issues.

The finding that SIPs too were not congruent is supported by previous studies suggesting that news and SIPs tend to convey different messages in their words and visuals (Cook, 1989; Hodes, 2007; Treichler, 1999). As to why this was the case, it does not seem plausible that these journalists and SIPs contributors used disagreeing verbal and visual frames strategically to impair memory for the words. Rather, this may have been due to the lack of congruent photos and hit-and-run decisions in an attempt to cope with the "tyranny of the empty frame" (Vobič & Tomanić Trivundža, 2015, p. 502). Also, the writer might not have had a say in the photo chosen to accompany his or her text. Finally, writers/editors may have not been interested in photos that did not go beyond the words—perceived as redundant.

Finally, the analysis of H10 revealed that the congruence ratio differed significantly by the frame conveyed. Specifically, the ratio was higher for the normal and carrier frames than for survivor and victim. This may be due to intention or lack of ability. If communicators want a frame to be clearly conveyed, they should invest in verbal-visual frame congruence. A communicator wanting to weaken the chance that an interpretation he or she disagrees with would be picked up by audiences may intentionally opt for inconsistency—as was perhaps the case in the example of the priest living with HIV/AIDS. Whatever the case, the finding that differences in the congruence ratio could be explained with reference to the verbal frame likely means that audiences will pick up some interpretations of PLWHA (normal, carrier) more clearly than others (survivor, victim). The potential implications of the frames were discussed at the beginning of this chapter.

These study results put forward that it is worthwhile to measure the extent to which the verbal frame in a given message matched the visual frame(s) in that message. Future studies could use the formula proposed here to calculate the congruence ratio between verbal frames and their visual counterparts. Scholars could further refine the formula to include prominence and dominance information (see Entman, 2004; Geise, Lobinger, & Brantner, 2013; Schwalbe, 2006). In this study, the verbal frame for each PLWHA was compared with the visual frame in each photo. Thus, the fact that some materials included one photo while others featured as many as 25 was taken into account. Future research could adjust the formula to account for the size of each photo relative to the space occupied by the accompanying words. But experimental research is needed first. Extrapolating from Matthes and Kohring (2008), it would seem that when a photo of Frankenstein is used to illustrate an article about biogenetics, the intended meaning is conveyed regardless of the size and placement of the photo.

Notes

1 This term was borrowed from Tuchman (1978, p. 1); it originally referred to news only.
2 A detailed history of HIV/AIDS is beyond my purpose. Interested readers are referred to alternative resources, such as AIDS.gov (2016), amfAR (2011), and Avert (2016).
3 Other than New Zealand, the United States is the only country in the world allowing pharmaceutical companies to advertise prescription drugs direct to consumers. Prescription drugs (short, Rx drugs) are those that are available only with a written prescription from a medical doctor. Most treatment options for HIV- and AIDS-related illnesses—known as antiretroviral medication—are prescription drugs (AIDSinfo, 2015).
4 This "sunny optimism" (Jones, 1997, p. 397) was not matched by the accompanying words. DTCA was shown to visually imply that taking the advertised medication would allow PLWHA to engage in strenuous physical activity (Jones, 1997; Klausner, Kim, & Kent, 2002; Scalvini, 2010). One prominent and much criticized example is a series of ads for Crixivan, a drug used in HIV treatment. There, humble slogans—such as "If you are HIV+, Crixivan may help you live a longer, healthier life"—were juxtaposed with hyperbolic photos showing gym-toned men rock-climbing.

Such visuals were criticized by the FDA, which requested more modest visuals. Obviously, equivalent verbal claims would be inadmissible. This lines up well with the argument that the "truth about advertising photography" is "that it does not necessarily describe the truth" (Garner, 2007, p. 191; see also Moriarty, 1987; Rosenblum, 1978).

Indeed, advertisers can more easily "hide" behind visual claims (Messaris, 1997; Messaris & Abraham, 2001), which are explicit enough to be understood by a reasonable percentage of the target audience but ambiguous enough to serve as a "shield of deniability" (Messaris & Abraham, 2001, p. 220). Advertisers criticized for making exaggerated visual claims can thus deny they had intended to convey the meaning picked up by the recipients (Craig, 1999; Khoury, 1997). This is because of the polysemy of visuals and their lack of an explicit propositional syntax, by which Messaris and Abraham (2001) mean that explicit claims are impossible through visuals.

5 In the *Introduction*, I distinguished between frames about issues and people. Investigating frames about the issue would have concerned the aspects of the diseases grouped under the label HIV/AIDS emphasized in verbal and visual communication. Scrutinizing frames about people, as I do here, involves studying the aspects of PLWHA's personalities and life stories that are selected and emphasized in a given message. I decided to focus on frames about people, known in the literature as character frames (Dan & Coleman, 2014; Grabe & Bucy, 2009). I offer the following reasons.

First, journalists and other communicators often put a face on dry topics in an attempt to involve audiences whose attention might otherwise not be engaged (Hong, 2012; Waters, McQueen, & Cameron, 2013; Zillmann & Brosius, 2000). This does not mean that personalized accounts have to be sympathetic toward the protagonists, as is the case in human-interest stories. Negative developments can also be personalized, as happens in crime news (Chibnall, 1977; Valentino, 1999). Illness-related topics often make people uncomfortable, perhaps because they force people to confront their own mortality (Kastenbaum, 2015). While HIV/AIDS may seem like a dry topic to those not immediately affected, personalized communication might engage many members of the audience.

Note that this high prevalence of personalized accounts is consequential. In the case of HIV/AIDS, this could mean that they can suppress base-rate or statistical information provided in that piece of communication (see Hastall & Knobloch-Westerwick, 2012; Knobloch-Westerwick & Sarge, 2015). This situation is known as base-rate fallacy (Ajzen, 1977; Bar-Hillel, 1980). The way people living with a certain medical condition are framed is a key component of the framing of the medical condition itself. This leads me to believe that these types of articles and PSAs contribute more to the framing of HIV/AIDS then nonpersonalized accounts.

For the group from which the protagonist was chosen, this is also important because audiences tend to make generalizations on the entire group based on the personalized account (Zillmann, 2006). Few of those directly affected would object when the coverage is positive, but negative accounts might court their resentment. This can lead to short-term priming effects. Gradual and cumulative effects are also conceivable when a certain type of framing recurs constantly (see Riles, Sangalang, Hurley, & Tewksbury, 2015; Stryker, 2008).

6 In my opinion, the constructs identified by Lupton (1999) are more fittingly described as character frames. Archetypes are stored in culture. When they are selected in communication and applied to a certain group of people, this

is, in my opinion, a framing act. Lupton's own definition of archetypes as "recurring patterns of representation and meaning" (p. 40) closely resembles that of frames.

7 This is perhaps due to the fact that the public expects local journalists to act as "good neighbors" (Poindexter, Heider, & McCombs, 2006, p. 77). In this way, local journalists attempt to cover issues immediately relevant to peoples' lives (Caburnay et al., 2003; Griffin & Dunwoody, 1995; Hamilton, 2004; Kaniss, 1991; Kim, Besley, Oh, & Kim, 2014). Health is certainly one of these issues.

The news media in general is interested in health-related topics because diseases fulfill most of the criteria for newsworthiness, in that they are novel or topical, potentially affect many people, are easy to put a face on, and allow the use of elite news sources (Armstrong, Carpenter, & Hojnacki, 2006; Gans, 1980).

8 www2.census.gov/geo/pdfs/maps-data/maps/reference/us_regdiv.pdf.

9 The following anecdote can illustrate the necessity of this step beyond the literature reviewed in Chapter 5. Early on, before having surveyed all the literature reviewed in Chapters 2 and 3, I hadn't put any thought in the way the data collection would have to be prepared. I had offered several lengthy sessions introducing student assistants to the codebook and was confident that the research instrument was clear and suitable for my purposes. Furthermore, I noticed that the student assistants were very vested into the project and worked with due diligence. Despite all this, reaching acceptable levels of intercoder reliability proved surprisingly difficult. The source of error proved to be the procedure: Having exposed coders to materials consisting of words *and* visuals, the text was coded consistently through the lens provided by the visuals. For instance, frame elements aligning with the survivor frame occurring in the text (i.e., strength, health, activism) were missed because the image suggested the carrier frame instead (i.e., deviance and dangerousness of PLWHA). One such article was about a former performer in adult films who contracted HIV before becoming an eloquent and vocal HIV/AIDS activist; it was illustrated with an older photo of the protagonist in a lascivious pose wearing see-through clothes and heavy makeup.

10 While David, Atun, Fille, and Monterola (2011) convincingly demonstrated that coding frames holistically (with just one variable) can be just as reliable as the coding of frames using multiple variables for the frame elements, these authors used coders with the same cultural background as the one from which their sample was drawn. But, as explained below in more depth, the students who coded the sample for this study—which was drawn from the United States—had a German background. Because of this, coding data holistically did not seem advisable.

11 They were as follows: problem definition, causal interpretation, treatment recommendation, and moral evaluation.

12 I could have chosen the more holistic ideological approach, but the fact that the symbolic-semiotic approach uses manifest categories that are then analyzed for their latent meaning seemed more suitable, given that my coders did not have a US background.

13 The other cues described in previous studies as suggestive of poor health (i.e., visible symptoms, signs of disease) did not surface in the subsample used for codebook development; the corresponding variables were thus excluded from the codebook. In fact, all photos encountered in the pretests showed asymptomatic, presentable individuals. This may be due to the wide availability of treatment today by comparison to the time when many of

the previous studies had been conducted. For this reason, I eliminated the variable measuring presentable appearance from the codebook, as—for my sample—it no longer seemed like a good criterion to point to various frames.

14 While I had considered all components proposed in previous research for inclusion in the visual codebook (see Table 3.1), not all of them could be kept. Specifically, "action" under power dynamics was dropped due to redundancy with "activity" and "position." Also, "overall appearance" was reduced to "mouth corners" which was more easily coded reliably. Finally, the "activity" category had to be adapted from politicians—who were investigated in the studies where this category was used—to PLWHA. Thus, activities like shaking hands were replaced by everyday activities and sports-related activities.

15 Coders did not collect data from the verbal and then from the visual component of the same articles and PSAs. Rather, the verbal counterpart of the visuals in one coder's sample was assigned to the other coder's sample.

16 The six variables measuring negative nonverbal behavior were aggregated for this purpose (e.g., downturned mouth corners, averted gaze, etc.). When at least half of the cues for nonverbal behavior were encountered, that individual's nonverbal behavior was considered negative. Submitting each of these variables individually to the reliability analysis with the variable measuring sickness-related props also returned very low alphas.

17 Due to their limited number, the observations for homosexual and bisexual PLWHA were collapsed into one category; this was also the case for observations for black/African American, Hispanic/Latino, Asian/Asian American PLWHA, and PLWHA of other races and ethnicities, which were collapsed into one "non-white" category.

18 See Chapter 5, Step 6 on how the verbal-visual frame congruence ratio was calculated.

7 Conclusion

Most messages investigated in our discipline consist of words and visuals. Limiting research to just one or the other is artificial and hinders our understanding of the nature of communication, the reasons behind it, and its potential effects.

This argument is as simple as it is compelling, which may be why so many researchers before me have advanced this line of reasoning. But if scholars accept the imperative of investigating words, visuals, and the interplay between them, then why do some communication scholars investigate just words, others just visuals, and very few the interplay?

I believe to have found the answer to this question in the paucity of methodological advice available. Thus, one of the goals pursued with this book was to address this shortcoming. Inspired by the social construction paradigm and intrigued by the idea that verbal and visual patterns of meaning are repeated over and over again in communication, I focused this effort on framing. Specifically, I aspired to facilitate integrative framing analyses in which researchers investigate verbal frames, visual frames, and the interplay between them.

I proposed that integrative framing analyses can be performed when a clearly defined sequence of steps is pursued. These steps guide the separation of the verbal and visual material for the collection of data and their reconnection for data analysis. A wide array of approaches for the identification of verbal frames on the one hand and visual frames on the other hand was reviewed in depth. I argued that each of the approaches had strengths and weaknesses. In principle scholars can choose among any of them to identify verbal and visual frames, respectively. I believe, however, that scholars should justify their decision with reference to theory (Entman, 1991, p. 8; Grittmann, 2013) and to effects studies (Entman, 2007, p. 168). To be precise, if current theorizing on framing provides sufficient support for the idea that a certain verbal or visual characteristic qualifies as a frame element, that element can be accounted for in content analyses. This support would come from previous effects studies showing that when alterations are made in that characteristic of a text or visual, there is a change in either the specific schema that gets activated in the mind of the audience or in the intensity

DOI: 10.4324/9781315171456-7

to which that schema seems applicable to the issue at hand. If no theoretical support exists, I believe that scholars should start with an effects study, making sure that all characteristics considered for inclusion in the content analysis are truly relevant to framing before actually conducting the content analysis.

Once the verbal and visual frames have been identified, they must be contrasted with each other. Quantitative studies can implement the formula I developed for determining the verbal-visual frame congruence ratio. Qualitative and critical studies can approach this comparison for each material in a sample with tools that suit their needs better than mathematics/statistics; a manual comparison or a comparison using software such as MAXQDA instead of SPSS may be the answer. Regardless of the preferred methodology, future studies are likely to bring about changes to the formula I proposed here for the measurement of the verbal-and-visual frame congruence ratio. For instance, aspects as story length or surface occupied by words and visuals, respectively, would have to be factored in. Also, the formula would have to be revised for the analysis of audiovisual material such as TV news or YouTube videos.

In this study, the congruence ratio was lowest for news. As news articles are, perhaps, the most typical object of investigation in communication studies, this result suggests that verbal-only or visual-only studies may not provide sufficient insight into the meanings audiences extract from news. Accordingly, I argue that researchers should analyze not just words, but also visuals, especially when they investigate news.

The proposal of an approach to integrative framing analysis was followed by the demonstration of each of its steps in an empirical study. To this end, the issue of HIV/AIDS was selected for study. More specifically, I investigated the frames conveyed for people living with HIV/AIDS (PLWHA) in news, special-interest publications, and public service announcements. I believe the findings obtained here improved our understanding of frames and framing.

One theoretical contribution that has been made was to provide support for the idea that frames are rather stable in time, as all verbal and visual frames the literature described for PLWHA since the 1980s were found in this study, which investigated material from 2013 to 2014. However, some differences were noticed between the frames as they were conveyed in the 1980s and the way they were conveyed in the 2010s. It seems that frames do change over time, little by little. The verbal frames identified in this study differed from those identified by others in one key aspect. Specifically, while previous literature suggested that the way a person contracted the virus would impact the frame used for that person, such was not the case in this study. In fact, information about the contagion scenario was scarce and typically nonjudgmental—that is, it was not presented in a way to suggest guilt/innocence, normality/deviance, and so on.

The visual frames were identified almost exclusively based on manifest content—what the people shown in the photos did, what props were used, and so forth. In this study, nonverbal behavior and structural features (i.e., latent meaning) barely played a role in the visual framing of PLWHA. (This was discussed at some length in the previous chapter.) From a theory-building perspective, it could be that nonverbal behavior and structural features do not qualify as frame elements. But such a conclusion would be premature. After all, previous research strongly suggested these characteristics are important in the framing of political news (Coleman & Wu, 2015; Grabe & Bucy, 2009). It is possible that the results obtained in this study merely suggest that the relevance of nonverbal behavior and structural features to visual framing is domain dependent.

Also, a methodological observation seems in order here. The verbal frames generally consisted of more elements than the visual frames. For instance, the verbal expression of the survivor frame included references to excellent health, excellent internal state, and activist work. Even though these characteristics point to different aspects of a person's life, they can be communicated coherently using words. Thus, using factor analyses, cluster analyses, or Cronbach's alpha to reveal which variables measure the same latent construct seems like a good idea for verbal frames.

However, compressing meaning ranging from health status, through internal state, to activist work into a single photo would be far more difficult. This would involve, for example, an athletic individual riding a bike while holding a banner or addressing a crowd at the same time. There are not many opportunities to take such a photo of a PLWHA. If visuals are very efficient in pointing directly to the objects/persons they depict, but at the same time are rather inefficient when elaborate propositions are to be made, then it may be that it takes several photos to convey complex meanings. Indeed, the three characteristics of visuals outlined by Messaris and Abraham (2001)—indexicality, analogical quality, and lack of propositional syntax—support this line of reasoning.

If this assumption is correct, this could mean that it is possible that completely different pictures (e.g., one showing a man biking in full gear and one showing a woman addressing a crowd from a stage) can convey the same frame even though these visual characteristics do not occur together in one photo. In other words, the question is as follows: Do audiences pick up the same frame from photos that are different in what they show? Moving forward, effects studies are needed to test this assumption. Perhaps small effects studies, or even just small pretests as known from experiments, can be conducted before researchers begin a content analysis. Choosing this two-step procedure would serve to validate such an approach. In a recent study, we exposed participants to images that differed in terms of content, but of which we expected that they would convey the same frame of PLWHA (Dan & Coleman, 2014). Participants generally agreed that all photos shown to them conveyed the same idea.

The differential use of frames in communication contexts and especially in newspapers sharing different characteristics suggest that not all frames are equally applied to PLWHA in all circumstances. From a theoretical viewpoint, this accentuates the idea of applicability in framing (Price & Tewksbury, 1997). Despite their enduring character, frames lose ground under some circumstances and gain ground under others. For instance, a few decades ago, homosexual people were often presented as deviant from the norm. While the deviant frame has not disappeared entirely from the cultural repertoire, it is now far less likely to be used in reference to this subpopulation. As Price and Tewksbury (1997) put it, audiences can change their views on whether or not a stored construct—the deviant frame—is applicable to the understanding of a certain issue or (group of) individual/s.

I would argue further that the differential use of frames in newspapers directed at audiences sharing different characteristics underscores the need for more diverse news samples than just the big metropolitan newspapers typically preferred by scholars. I understand that scholars may be more interested in national news than in local news, but given differences in the types of stories deemed relevant for coverage and the way they are covered (see Franklin & Parry, 1998; Gans, 2003; Kaniss, 1991), I would argue audiences' high interest in local news (Coulson, Lacy, & Wilson, 2000; Mitchell, 2014) would have to be considered when researchers decide on what constitutes an appropriate sample. When scholars analyze local news, they might also include local advocacy materials in their study. Contrasting frames in news stories and frames in advocacy materials in the same study can provide superior understanding of the environment in which news frames emerged.

Another theoretical contribution made here concerns the investigation of frame building, an area that has been severely neglected in previous research (Borah, 2011). I argue that the intention to understand where news frames come from—be they verbal or visual—should be at the core of every news framing analysis (see also Reese, 2007). Having found similarities between news frames and advocacy frames and given the significant differences discovered between verbal news frames and news sources, and especially between visual news frames and photo sources, this study illustrated how rewarding this effort can be. It is my hope that the results obtained here will motivate more scholars to conduct this type of research.

Despite the object of investigation chosen for this study, it seems important to emphasize that my approach to integrative framing analysis is not limited to character frames, to the topic of HIV/AIDS, or to the area of health communication. It can be applied to any other object of investigation, provided it consists of both words and visuals.

It is my firm belief that a wide recognition of the merits and an increased acceptance of the need for integrative studies is within reach. I hope this book revealed ways in which scholars familiar with verbal analyses can collaborate with visual researchers to achieve a better understanding of messages consisting of both words and visuals. After successfully spotlighting visual research, framing can also fuel integrative studies. Such integrative studies might become emblematic for communication studies and set our discipline apart from other social sciences, thus helping it become "a master discipline" (see Entman, 1993, p. 51).

Without a doubt, it will take time for integrative analyses to become the norm. In my view, this development is imminent, and the research results obtained justify the additional effort.

References

Aday, S., Cluverius, J., & Livingston, S. (2005). As goes the statue, so goes the war: The emergence of the victory frame in television coverage of the Iraq war. *Journal of Broadcasting & Electronic Media*, *49*(3), 314–331.

Adoni, H., & Mane, S. (1984). Media and the social construction of reality: Toward an integration of theory and research. *Communication Research*, *11*(3), 323–340. doi:10.1177/009365084011003001.

Aggleton, P., & Parker, R. (2002). *HIV/AIDS stigma and discrimination: A conceptual framework and basis for action*. Geneva: UNAIDS.

AIDS.gov. (2016). A timeline of HIV/AIDS. Retrieved from https://aids.gov/hiv-aids-basics/hiv-aids-101/aids-timeline/.

AIDSinfo. (2015). HIV treatment. FDA-Approved HIV Medicines. Retrieved from https://aidsinfo.nih.gov/education-materials/fact-sheets/21/58/fda-approved-hiv-medicines.

Ajzen, I. (1977). Intuitive theories of events and the effects of base-rate information on prediction. *Journal of Personality and Social Psychology*, *35*(5), 303–314.

Albert, E. (1986). Illness and deviance: The response of the press to AIDS. In D. A. Feldman & T. M. Johnson (Eds.), *The social dimensions of AIDS: Method and theory* (pp. 163–178). New York: Praeger.

Albert, E. (1989). AIDS and the press: The creation and transformation of a social problem. In J. Best (Ed.), *Images of issues: Typifying contemporary social problems* (pp. 39–54). Hawthorne, NY: Aldine de Gruyter.

Alonzo, A. A., & Reynolds, N. R. (1995). Stigma, HIV and AIDS: An exploration and elaboration of a stigma trajectory. *Social Science & Medicine*, *41*(3), 303–315. doi:10.1016/0277-9536(94)00384-6.

Andsager, J. L., & Smiley, L. (1998). Evaluating the public information: Shaping news coverage of the silicone implant controversy. *Public Relations Review*, *24*(2), 183–201. doi:10.1016/s0363-8111(99)80050-2.

Armstrong, E. M., Carpenter, D. P., & Hojnacki, M. (2006). Whose deaths matter? Mortality, advocacy, and attention to disease in the mass media. *Journal of Health Politics, Policy and Law*, *31*(4), 729–772.

Arroyave, J. (2012). Health, news, and media information. In R. Obregon & S. Waisbord (Eds.), *The handbook of global health communication* (pp. 194–214). Malden, MA: Wiley-Blackwell.

Avert. (2016). History of HIV and AIDS Overview. Retrieved from www.avert.org/professionals/history-hiv-aids/overview.

Baerns, B. (1979). Öffentlichkeitsarbeit als Determinante journalistischer Informationsleistungen. Thesen zur realistischen Beschreibung von Medieninhalten [Public relations as a determinant of journalists' information services. Theses on the realistic description of media content]. *Publizistik*, *24*(3), 301–331.
Baerns, B. (1991). *Öffentlichkeitsarbeit oder Journalismus? Zum Einfluss im Mediensystem [Public Relations or Journalism? On Influence in the Media System]*. Cologne: Verlag Wissenschaft und Politik.
Baker, A. (1986). The portrayal of AIDS in the media: An analysis of articles in the New York Times. In D. Feldmans & T. Johnson (Eds.), *The social dimensions of AIDS* (pp. 179–194). New York: Praeger.
Banning, S., & Coleman, R. (2009). Louder than words: A content analysis of presidential candidates' televised nonverbal communication. *Visual Communication Quarterly*, *16*(1), 4–17.
Bardhan, N. (2001). Transnational AIDS-HIV news narratives: A critical exploration of overarching frames. *Mass Communication and Society*, *4*(3), 283–309.
Bardhan, N. (2002). Accounts from the field: A public relations perspective on global AIDS/HIV. *Journal of Health Communication*, *7*(3), 221–244.
Baresch, B., Hsu, S., & Reese, S. D. (2012). The power of framing: New challenges for researching the structure of meaning in news. In S. Allan (Ed.), *Routledge companion to news and journalism studies* (pp. 637–647). New York: Routledge.
Bar-Hillel, M. (1980). The base-rate fallacy in probability judgments. *Acta Psychologica*, *44*(3), 211–233. doi:10.1016/0001-6918(80)90046-3.
Barlow, T., & Wogalter, M. S. (1993). Alcoholic beverage warnings in magazine and television advertisements. *Journal of Consumer Research*, *20*(1), 147–156.
Barnett, B. (2003). Guilty and threatening: Visual bias in television news crime stories. *Journalism & Communication Monographs*, *5*(3), 103–155.
Barnhurst, K. G., Vari, M., & Rodriguez, I. (2004). Mapping visual studies in communication. *Journal of Communication*, *45*(4), 616–644.
Barry, A. M. (2005). Perception theory. In K. Smith, S. Moriarty, G. Barbatsis, & K. Kenney (Eds.), *Handbook of visual communication: Theory, methods, and media* (pp. 45–62). Mahwah, NJ: Lawrence Erlbaum.
Barthelson, M. (2002). *Behaviour in online news reading*, Lund University. Retrieved from http://lup.lub.lu.se/luur/download?func=downloadFile&recordOId=1329001&fileOId=1329002.
Barthes, R. (1981). *Camera lucida: Reflections on photography*. New York: Hill and Wang.
Bartholomé, G., Lecheler, S., & de Vreese, C. H. (2015). Manufacturing conflict? How journalists intervene in the conflict frame building process. *The International Journal of Press/Politics*, *20*(4), 438–457. doi:10.1177/1940161215595514.
Bates, A. E. (2007). Wearing the T-shirt: An exploration of the ideological underpinnings of visual representations of the African body with HIV or AIDS. *African Journal of AIDS Research*, *6*(1), 67–78.
Becker, H. S. (1995). Visual sociology, documentary photography, and photojournalism: It's (almost) all a matter of context. *Visual Sociology*, *1–2*, 5–14.
Bedingfield, S., & Anshari, D. (2014). Thinking about Romney: Frame building in a battleground state in the 2012 presidential election. *Journalism & Mass Communication Quarterly*, *91*(1), 78–97. doi:10.1177/1077699013514417.

Bell, P. (2001). Content analysis of visual images. In T. Van Leeuwen & C. Jewitt (Eds.), *Handbook of visual analysis* (pp. 10–34). Thousand Oaks, CA: Sage.

Bell, P., & Milic, M. (2002). Goffman's gender advertisement revisited: Combining content analysis with semiotic analysis. *Visual Communication*, *1*(2), 203–222.

Benford, R. D., & Snow, D. A. (2000). Framing processes and social movements: An overview and assessment. *Annual Review of Sociology*, *26*(1), 611–639.

Bennett, W. L. (1990). Toward a theory of press-state relations in the United States. *Journal of Communication*, *40*(2), 103–125.

Bennett, W. L. (2005). *News: The politics of illusion* (6th ed.). New York: Longman.

Bennett, W. L., Lawrence, R. G., & Livingston, S. (2006). None dare call it torture: Indexing and the limits of press independence in the Abu Ghraib scandal. *Journal of Communication*, *56*(3), 467–485.

Bentele, G., Liebert, T., & Seeling, S. (1997). Von der Determination zur Intereffikation. Ein integriertes Modell zum Verhältnis von Public Relations und Journalismus [From determination to intereffication. An integrated model for the relationship between public relations and journalism]. In G. Bentele & M. Haller (Eds.), *Aktuelle Entstehung von Öffentlichkeit. Akteure-Strukturen-Veränderungen* (Vol. 24, pp. 225–250). Constance: UVK.

Berger, A. A. (1981). Semiotics and TV. In R. R. Adler (Ed.), *Understanding television: Essays on television as a social and cultural force* (pp. 91–114). New York: Praeger.

Berger, M. (1992). *How art becomes history: Essays on art, society, and culture in post-new deal America*. New York: Harper Collins.

Berger, A. A. (1995). *Cultural criticism: A primer of key concepts*. Thousand Oaks, CA: Sage.

Berger, P. L., & Luckmann, T. (1967). *The social construction of reality: A treatise in the sociology of knowledge*. London: Penguin.

Bergstroem, B. (2008). *Essentials of visual communication*. London: Thames & Hudson.

Berkowitz, D. (1987). TV news sources and news channels: A study in agenda building. *Journalism & Mass Communication Quarterly*, *64*(2/3), 508–513.

Berkowitz, D. (1991). Assessing forces in the selection of local television news. *Journal of Broadcasting & Electronic Media*, *35*(2), 245–251.

Berkowitz, D., & Adams, D. B. (1990). Information subsidy and agenda building in local television news. *Journalism Quarterly*, *67*(4), 723–731.

Berres, I. (2014). Verstrickungen von Ärzten mit der Industrie: Finanzielle Interessenkonflikte recherchieren und bewerten [Entanglements of physicians with industry: Researching and evaluating financial conflicts of interest]. In V. Lilienthal, D. Reineck, & T. Schnedler (Eds.), *Qualität im Gesundheitsjournalismus. Perspektiven aus Wissenschaft und Praxis* (pp. 265–284). Wiesbaden: SpringerVS.

Biddle, N., Conte, L., & Diamond, E. (1993). AIDS in the media: Entertainment or infotainment. In S. C. Ratzan (Ed.), *AIDS: Effective health communication for the 90s* (pp. 113–140). Washington, DC: Taylor & Francis.

Bilandzic, H. (2008). Triangulation. In W. Donsbach (Ed.), *The international encyclopedia of communication*. Blackwell Reference Online: Blackwell Publishing. Retrieved from www.communicationencyclopedia.com/subscriber/tocnode.html?id=g9781405131995_yr2015_chunk_g978140513199525_ss60-1.

Biocca, F. (2014). The role of communication codes in political ads. In F. Biocca (Ed.), *Television and political advertising: Volume II: Signs, codes, and images* (pp. 27–43). New York: Routledge.

Bird, S. E., & Dardenne, R. W. (1988). Myth, chronicle, and story: Exploring the narrative qualities of news. In J. W. Carey (Ed.), *Media, myths, and narratives: Television and the press* (Vol. 15, pp. 67–86). Thousand Oaks, CA: Sage.

Blum, J., & Bucher, H.-J. (1998). *Die Zeitung: Ein Multimedium. Textdesign-ein Gestaltungskonzept für Text, Bild und Grafik [The newspaper: A multi-medium. Text design—A design concept for text, image and graphics]*. Constance: UVK.

Blumler, J. G., & Gurevitch, M. (1995). *The crisis of public communication*. London: Routledge.

Bock, M. A., & Araiza, J. A. (2015). Facing the death penalty while facing the cameras. *Journalism Practice*, *9*(3), 314–331. doi:10.1080/17512786.2014.964496.

Bock, A., Isermann, H., & Knieper, T. (2012). Quantitative content analysis of the visual. In J. Hughes (Ed.), *Sage visual methods* (Vol. III: Interpretation and Classification, pp. 313–334). Thousand Oaks, CA: Sage.

Boesman, J., d'Haenens, L., & Van Gorp, B. (2016). Between silence and salience: A multimethod model to study frame building from a journalistic perspective. *Communication Methods and Measures*, *10*(4), 233–247. doi:10.1080/19312458.2016.1228864.

Bohan, J. (1996). *The psychology of sexual orientation: Coming to terms*. New York: Routledge.

Borah, P. (2009). Comparing visual framing in newspapers: Hurricane Katrina versus Tsunami. *Newspaper Research Journal*, *30*(1), 50–57.

Borah, P. (2011). Conceptual issues in framing theory: A systematic examination of a decade's literature. *Journal of Communication*, *61*(2), 246–263. doi:10.1111/j.1460-2466.2011.01539.x.

Brandenburg, H. (2002). Who follows whom? The impact of parties on media agenda formation in the 1997 British general election campaign. *Harvard International Journal of Press/Politics*, *7*(3), 34–54.

Brier, J. (2009). *Infectious ideas: US political responses to the AIDS crisis*. Chapel Hill, NC: University of North Carolina Press.

Brosius, H.-B. (1993). The effects of emotional pictures in television news. *Communication Research*, *20*(1), 105–124.

Brüggemann, M. (2014). Between frame setting and frame sending: How journalists contribute to news frames. *Communication Theory*, *24*(1), 61–82. doi:10.1111/comt.12027.

Bryant, J., & Davies, J. (2008). Selective exposure. In W. Donsbach (Ed.), *The international encyclopedia of communication*. Blackwell Reference Online: Blackwell Publishing. Retrieved from www.communicationencyclopedia.com/subscriber/tocnode.html?id=g9781405131995_yr2015_chunk_g978140513199524_ss27-1.

Bucher, H.-J. (2008). Vergleichende Rezeptionsforschung: Theorien, Methoden, Befunde [Comparative effects studies: Theories, methods, findings]. In G. Melischek, J. Seethaler, & J. Wilke (Eds.), *Medien & Kommunikationsforschung im Vergleich. Grundlagen, Gegenstandsbereiche, Verfahrensweisen* (pp. 309–340). Wiesbaden: VS.

Bucher, H.-J., & Schumacher, P. (2006). The relevance of attention for selecting news content. An eye-tracking study on attention patterns in the reception of print and online media. *Communications: The European Journal of Communication Research*, *31*(3), 347–368.

Bucy, E. P., & Newhagen, J. E. (1999). The emotional appropriateness heuristic: Processing televised presidential reactions to the news. *Journal of Communication*, *49*(4), 59–79.

Burgoon, J. K., Buller, D. B., & Woodall, W. G. (1996). *Nonverbal communication: The unspoken dialogue*. New York: McGraw-Hill.

Busselle, R., & Bhandzic, H. (2011). Images in readers' construction of news narratives. In S. D. Ross & P. M. Lester (Eds.), *Images that injure: Pictorial stereotypes in the media* (3rd ed., pp. 31–42). Santa Barbara, CA: Praeger.

Butler, O. (2007). Narrative, documentary, and editorial photography. In M. R. Peres (Ed.), *The focal encyclopedia of photography. Digital imaging, theory and applications, history, and science* (4th ed., pp. 334–336). Boston, MA: Focal Press.

Caburnay, C. A., Kreuter, M. W., Luke, D. A., Logan, R. A., Jacobsen, H. A., Reddy, V. C., ... Zayed, H. R. (2003). Health behavior: Coverage of diet, activity, and tobacco in local newspapers. *Health Education Behavior*, *30*(6), 709–722.

Callaghan, K., & Schnell, F. (2001). Assessing the democratic debate: How the news media frame elite policy discourse. *Political Communication*, *18*(2), 183–212.

Cameron, G., & Lee, C. M. (2006). *Does involvement moderate the effectiveness of gain versus loss framed messages alone?* Paper presented at the Annual Meeting of the International Communication Association (ICA), Dresden, Germany.

Campbell, D. (2008). *The visual economy of HIV/AIDS*. Brooklyn, NY: AIDS, Security and Conflict Initiative.

Campbell, C., Foulis, C. A., Maimane, S., & Sibiya, Z. (2005). "I have an evil child at my house": Stigma and HIV/AIDS management in a South African community. *American Journal of Public Health*, *95*(5), 808–815.

Cappella, J., Leader, A., Kang, Y., & White, K. (2007). *A rating scale for visual-verbal redundancy in antismoking video ads: Reliability and validity*. Paper presented at the Annual Meeting of the International Communication Association, San Francisco, CA.

Carragee, K. M., & Roefs, W. (2004). The neglect of power in recent framing research. *Journal of Communication*, *54*(2), 214–233.

Carter, R. F., Stamm, K. R., & Heintz-Knowles, K. (1992). Agenda setting and consequentiality. *Journalism Quarterly*, *69*(4), 868–877.

Centers for Disease Control [CDC]. (1981). *MMWR: Morbidity and Mortality Weekly Report*, *30*(21).

Centers for Disease Control and Prevention [CDC]. (2013a). HIV cost-effectiveness. Retrieved from www.cdc.gov/hiv/prevention/ongoing/costeffectiveness/.

Centers for Disease Control and Prevention [CDC]. (2013b). HIV in the United States: At a glance. Retrieved from www.cdc.gov/hiv/pdf/statistics_basics_factsheet.pdf.

Centers for Disease Control and Prevention [CDC]. (2013c). *HIV surveillance report. Diagnoses of HIV infection in the United States and dependent areas,*

2011 (Vol. 23). Atlanta, GA: National Center for HIV/AIDS, Viral Hepatitis, STD, and TB Prevention. Division of HIV/AIDS Prevention.
Centers for Disease Control and Prevention [CDC]. (2015a). HIV/AIDS. Retrieved from www.cdc.gov/hiv/.
Centers for Disease Control and Prevention [CDC]. (2015b). Living with HIV: Treatment. Retrieved from www.cdc.gov/hiv/basics/livingwithhiv/treatment.html.
Chang, C. (2013). Seeing is believing: The direct and contingent influence of pictures in health promotion advertising. *Health Communication*, *28*(8), 822–834. doi:10.1080/10410236.2012.726403.
Chen, S., & Chaiken, S. (1999). The heuristic-systematic model in its broader context. In S. Chen & Y. Trope (Eds.), *Dual-process theories in social psychology* (pp. 73–96). New York: Guilford.
Chibnall, S. (1977). *Law-and-order: An analysis of crime reporting in the British press*. London: Tavistock.
Clarke, J. N. (1992). Cancer, heart disease, and AIDS: What do the media tell us about these diseases? *Health Communication*, *4*, 105–120.
Clarke, J. N., & Binns, J. (2006). The portrayal of heart disease in mass print magazines 1991–2001. *Health Communication*, *19*(1), 39–48.
Clarke, J. N., McLellan, L., & Hoffman-Goetz, L. (2006). The portrayal of HIV/AIDS in two popular African American magazines. *Journal of Health Communication*, *11*(5), 495–507.
Clawson, R. A., Strine, H. C. N. I., & Waltenburg, E. N. (2003). Framing supreme court decisions: The mainstream versus the black press. *Journal of Black Studies*, *33*(6), 784–800. doi:10.2307/3180846.
Cochran, W. G. (1954). Some methods of strengthening the common chi-square tests. *Biometrics*, *10*(4), 417–451.
Cohen, J. (1988). *Statistical power analysis for the behavioral sciences* (2nd ed.). Hillsdale, NJ: Lawrence Erlbaum.
Coleman, C.-L. (1995). Science, technology and risk coverage of a community conflict. *Media, Culture & Society*, *17*(1), 65–79.
Coleman, R. (2010). Framing the pictures in our heads. Exploring the framing and agenda-setting effects of visual images. In P. D'Angelo & J. A. Kuypers (Eds.), *Doing news framing analysis* (pp. 233–261). New York: Routledge.
Coleman, R., & Hatley Major, L. (2014). Ethical health communication: A content analysis of predominant frames and primes in public service announcements. *Journal of Mass Media Ethics*, *29*(2), 91–107. doi:10.1080/08900523.2014.893773.
Coleman, R., & Wasike, B. (2004). Visual elements in public journalism newspapers in an election: A content analysis of the photographs and graphics in campaign 2000. *Journal of Communication*, *54*(3), 456–473.
Coleman, R., & Wu, H. D. (2015). *Image and emotion in voter decisions. The affect agenda*. Lanham, MD: Lexington Books.
Conrad, P. (1999). Uses of expertise: Sources, quotes and voices in the reporting of genetics in the news. *Public Understanding of Science*, *8*(4), 285–302.
Cook, T. E. (1989). *Setting the record straight: The construction of homosexuality on television news*. Paper presented at the Inside/Outside Conference of the Lesbian and Gay Studies Center, New Haven, CT.
Cook, T. E., & Colby, D. E. (1992). The mass-mediated epidemic: The politics of AIDS on the nightly network news. In E. Fee & D. M. Fox (Eds.),

AIDS: The making of a chronic sisease (pp. 84–122). Berkeley: University of California Press.

Corbett, J. B., & Mori, M. (1999). Medicine, media, and celebrities: News coverage of breast cancer, 1960–1995. *Journalism & Mass Communication Quarterly*, *76*(2), 229–249.

Corfe, R. (2008). *Egalitarianism of the free society: And the end of class conflict*. Bury: Arena Books.

Coulson, M. (2004). Attributing emotion to static body postures: Recognition, accuracy, confusions and viewpoint dependence. *Journal of Nonverbal Behavior*, *28*(2), 117–139.

Coulson, D. C., Lacy, S., & Wilson, J. (2000). *Weekly newspaper industry: A baseline study*. Paper presented at the Annual Conference of the Association for Education in Journalism and Mass Communication, Phoenix, AZ.

Craig, R. (1999). Fact, public opinion and persuasion: The rise of the visual in journalism and advertising. In B. Brennen & H. Hardt (Eds.), *Picturing the past: Media, history and photography* (pp. 36–59). Urbana, IL: University of Illinois Press.

Crimp, D. (1988). How to have promiscuity in an epidemic. In D. Crimp (Ed.), *AIDS: Cultural analysis, cultural activism* (pp. 237–273). Cambridge, MA: MIT Press.

Crimp, D. (1992). Portraits of people with AIDS. In L. Grossberg, C. Nelson, & P. Treichler (Eds.), *Cultural studies* (pp. 117–133). New York: Routledge.

Cullen, T., & Callaghan, R. (2010). Reporting HIV in Papua New Guinea: Trends and omissions from 2000 to 2010. *Pacific Journalism Review*, *16*(2), 163–177.

Dahlgren, P. (2008). Television news, visual components of. In W. Donsbach (Ed.), *The international encyclopedia of communication*. Blackwell Reference Online: Blackwell Publishing. Retrieved from www.communicationencyclopedia.com/subscriber/tocnode.html?id=g9781405131995_chunk_g978140513199525_ss39-1.

Dahmen, N. S. (2009). Snowflake white and politically right: Photographic framing in news media coverage of stem cell research. *Visual Communication Quarterly*, *16*(1), 18–31.

Dan, V. (2015). Patientengerichtete Werbung für verschreibungspflichtige Medikamente (DTCA)-Überblick und Forschungslücken [Direct-to-consumer advertising for pharmaceutical products (DTCA)—A literature review and directions for future research]. In M. Schäfer, O. Quiring, C. Rossmann, M. Hastall, & E. Baumann (Eds.), *Gesundheitskommunikation im gesellschaftlichen Wandel: Chancen und Herausforderungen* (pp. 63–73). Baden-Baden: Nomos.

Dan, V. (2018, in press). Empirical and non-empirical methods. In J. Matthes, R. Potter, & C. S. Davis (Eds.), *Wiley international encyclopedia of communication research methods*. Hoboken, NJ: Wiley.

Dan, V., & Coleman, R. (2014). *Coming down from the ivory tower: Visual frames of HIV/AIDS in the academic literature and broader society*. Paper presented at the 64th Annual Conference of the International Communication Association, Seattle, WA.

Dan, V., & Ihlen, Ø. (2011a). Framing expertise. A cross-cultural analysis of success in framing contests. *Journal of Communication Management*, *15*(4), 368–388.

Dan, V., & Ihlen, Ø. (2011b). *Towards the empirical assessment of complex frames: A method for combining analysis of verbal and visual elements.* Paper presented at the 61st Annual Conference of the International Communication Association, Boston, MA.
Dan, V., & Iorgoveanu, A. (2013). Still on the beaten path: How gender impacted the coverage of male and female romanian candidates for European office. *International Journal of Press/Politics*, *18*(2), 208–233. doi:10.1177/1940161212473508.
D'Angelo, P., & Kuypers, J. A. (2010). Introduction-doing news framing analysis. In P. D'Angelo & J. A. Kuypers (Eds.), *Doing news framing analysis: Empirical and theoretical perspectives* (pp. 1–13). New York: Routledge.
David, P. (2008). Dual coding theory. In W. Donsbach (Ed.), *The international encyclopedia of communication*. Blackwell Reference Online: Blackwell Publishing. Retrieved from www.communicationencyclopedia.com/subscriber/tocnode.html?id=g9781405131995_chunk_g97814051319959_ss68-1.
David, C. C., Atun, J. M., Fille, E., & Monterola, C. (2011). Finding frames: Comparing two methods of frame analysis. *Communication Methods and Measures*, *5*(4), 329–351. doi:10.1080/19312458.2011.624873.
Dearing, J., & Rogers, E. (1996). *Agenda-setting*. Thousand Oaks, CA: Sage.
DeJong, W., Wolf, R. C., & Austin, S. B. (2001). U.S. Federally funded television public service announcements (PSAs) to prevent HIV/AIDS: A content analysis. *Journal of Health Communication*, *6*(3), 249–263. doi:10.1080/108107301752384433.
Denzin, N. K. (2009). *The research act: A theoretical introduction to sociological methods* (4th ed.). London: Aldine Transaction.
DeSilva, M., Muskavitch, M. A. T., & Roche, J. P. (2004). Print media coverage of antibiotic resistance. *Science Communication*, *26*(1), 31–43.
de Souza, R. (2007). The construction of HIV/AIDS in indian newspapers: A frame analysis. *Health Communication*, *21*(3), 257–266.
Devine, P. G., Plant, E. A., & Harrison, K. (1999). The problem of "us" versus "them" and AIDS stigma. *American Behavioral Scientist*, *42*(7), 1212–1228.
de Vreese, C. H. (2003). *Framing Europe: Television news and European integration*. Amsterdam: Aksant.
de Vreese, C. H. (2005). News framing: Theory and typology. *Information Design Journal + Document Design*, *13*(51–62).
de Vreese, C. H. (2010). Framing the economy: Effects of journalistic news frames. In P. D'Angelo & J. A. Kuypers (Eds.), *Doing news framing analysis: Empirical and theoretical perspectives* (pp. 187–214). New York: Routledge.
de Vreese, C. H., & Lecheler, S. (2012). News framing research: An overview and new developments. In H. A. Semetko & M. Scammell (Eds.), *The sage handbook of political communication* (pp. 292–307). Thousand Oaks, CA: Sage.
Dhooper, S. S., & Royse, D. D. (1989). Rural attitudes about AIDS: A statewide survey. *Human Services in the Rural Environment*, *13*(1), 17–22.
Dimitrova, D. V., & Kostadinova, P. (2013). Identifying antecedents of the strategic game frame: A longitudinal analysis. *Journalism & Mass Communication Quarterly*, *90*(1), 75–88.
Dimitrova, D. V., & Strömbäck, J. (2012). Election news in Sweden and the United States: A comparative study of sources and media frames. *Journalism*, *13*(5), 604–619.

Dixon, G. N., McKeever, B. W., Holton, A. E., Clarke, C., & Eosco, G. (2015). The power of a picture: Overcoming scientific misinformation by communicating weight-of-evidence information with visual exemplars. *Journal of Communication*, *65*(4), 639–659. doi:10.1111/jcom.12159.

Doka, K. J. (1997). *AIDS, fear and society: Challenging the dreaded disease*. London: Taylor & Francis.

Donohue, G. A., Tichenor, P. J., & Olien, C. N. (1973). Mass media functions, knowledge and social control. *Journalism Quarterly*, *50*, 652–659.

Donohue, G. A., Tichenor, P. J., & Olien, C. N. (1995). A guard dog perspective on the role of the media. *Journal of Communication*, *45*, 115–132.

Donsbach, W. (1991). *Medienwirkung trotz Selektion. Einflußfaktoren auf die Zuwendung zu Zeitungsinhalten [Media effects despite selection. Factors influencing attention to newspaper content]*. Vienna, Austria: Böhlau.

Donsbach, W., & Meißner, A. (2004). PR und Nachrichtenagenturen. Missing link in der kommunikationswissenschaftlichen Forschung [PR and news agencies. Missing link in communication studies]. In J. Raupp & J. Klewes (Eds.), *Quo vadis Public Relations? Auf dem Weg zum Kommunikationsmanagement: Bestandsaufnahme und Entwicklungen [Quo vadis public relations? On the path toward communication management: appraisal and developments]* (pp. 113–124). Wiesbaden, Germany: VS.

Dotson, D. M., Jacobson, S. K., Kaid, L. L., & Carlton, J. S. (2012). Media coverage of climate change in Chile: A content analysis of conservative and liberal newspapers. *Environmental Communication*, *6*(1), 64–81. doi:10.1080/17524032.2011.642078.

Drew, D. G., & Grimes, T. (1987). Audio-visual redundancy and TV news recall. *Communication Research*, *14*(4), 452–461.

Drueilhe, E. (1988). *Mortal embrace: Living with AIDS*. New York: Hill and Wang.

D'Silva, M. U., Leichty, G., & Agarwal, V. (2011). Cultural representations of HIV/AIDS in indian print media. *Intercultural Communication Studies*, *20*(2), 75–88.

Durham, F. S. (1998). News frames as social narratives: TWA flight 800. *Journal of Communication*, *48*(4), 100–117. doi:10.1111/j.1460-2466.1998.tb02772.x.

Dutta, M. J. (2014). Culture-centered approaches. In T. L. Thompson (Ed.), *Encyclopedia of health communication* (pp. 284–290). Thousand Oaks, CA: Sage.

Eder, J. (2002). Aufmerksamkeit ist keine Selbstverständlichkeit. Eine Diskurskritik und ein Klärungsvorschlag [Attention is not self-evident. A criticism of discourse and a proposal for clarification]. In K. Hickethier & J. K. Bleicher (Eds.), *Aufmerksamkeit, Medien und Ökonomie [Attention, media and economy]* (pp. 15–47). Hamburg: LIT.

Ehrenreich, B. (2010). *Smile or die: How positive thinking fooled America and the world*. London: Granta Books.

Elliott, D. (2011). Ethical responsibilities and the power of pictures. In S. D. Ross & P. M. Lester (Eds.), *Images that injure: Pictorial stereotypes in the media* (3rd ed., pp. 9–19). Santa Barbara, CA: Praeger.

Emmison, M., & Smith, P. (2012). Putting visual data into focus. In J. Hughes (Ed.), *Sage visual methods* (Vol. I: Principles, Issues, Debates and Controversies in Visual Research, pp. 145–166). Thousand Oaks, CA: Sage.

Entman, R. M. (1991). Framing U.S. coverage of international news: Contrasts in narratives of the KAL and Iran air incidents. *Journal of Communication, 41*(4), 6–27.

Entman, R. M. (1993). Framing: Toward clarification of a fractured paradigm. *Journal of Communication, 43*(4), 51–58.

Entman, R. M. (2003). Cascading activation: Contesting the White House's frame after 9/11. *Political Communication, 20*(4), 415–432.

Entman, R. M. (2004). *Projections of power: Framing news, public opinion, and U.S. foreign policy.* Chicago, IL: University of Chicago Press.

Entman, R. M. (2007). Framing bias: Media in the distribution of power. *Journal of Communication, 57*(1), 163–173.

Entman, R. M., Matthes, J., & Pellicano, L. (2008). Nature, sources and effects of news framing. In K. Wahl-Jorgensen & T. Hanitzsch (Eds.), *The handbook of journalism studies* (pp. 175–190). New York: Routledge.

Entwistle, V., & Williams, B. (2008). Health literacy: The need to consider images as well as words. *Health Expectations, 11*(2), 99–101.

Ericson, R. V., Baranek, P. M., & Chan, J. B. L. (1989). *Negotiating control: A study of news sources.* Milton Keynes: Open University Press.

Evensen, D. T., & Clarke, C. E. (2012). Efficacy information in media coverage of infectious disease risks: An ill predicament? *Science Communication, 34*(3), 392–418.

Faden, R. R., & Faden, A. I. (1978). The ethics of health education as public health policy. *Health Education Monographs,* 6, 180–197.

Fahmy, S. (2004a). *Framing visual news: The 9/11 attack & the war in Afghanistan in English- and Arabic-language newspapers.* Paper presented at the Annual Meeting of the International Communication Association, New Orleans, LA.

Fahmy, S. (2004b). Picturing Afghan women: A content analysis of AP wire photographs during the Taliban regime and after the fall of the Taliban regime. *Gazette, 66*(2), 91–112. doi:10.1177/0016549204041472.

Fahmy, S. (2007). "They Took It Down": Exploring determinants of visual reporting in the toppling of the Saddam statue in national and international newspapers. *Mass Communication and Society, 10*(2), 143–170.

Fahmy, S., & Kim, D. (2008). Picturing the Iraq war: Constructing the image of war in the british and US press. *Gazette, 70*(6), 443–462. doi:10.1177/1748048508096142.

Fahmy, S., Bock, M. A., & Wanta, W. (2014). *Visual communication theory and research. A mass communication perspective.* New York: Palgrave Macmillan.

Fairclough, N. (1995). *Media Discourse.* New York: St. Martin.

Findlay, J. M., & Gilchrist, I. D. (2003). *Active vision. The psychology of looking and seeing.* Oxford, MA: Oxford University Press.

Finn, J. M. (2009). *Capturing the criminal image: From mug shot to surveillance society.* Minneapolis: University of Minnesota Press.

Fiske, J. (2011). *Television culture* (2nd ed.). London: Routledge.

Fitzgerald, M. (1997). Local TV news lacks substance (nationwide study of television news). *Editor and Publisher, 130*(21), 8–10.

Franklin, B., & Parry, J. (1998). Old habits die hard: Journalism's changing professional commitments and local newspaper reporting of the 1997 general election. In B. Franklin & D. Murphy (Eds.), *Making the local news: Local journalism in context* (pp. 209–227). London: Routledge.

Freud, S. (1952). *On dreams*. New York: Norton.

Frisch, A.-L., Camerini, L., & Schulz, P. J. (2012). The impact of presentation style on the retention of online health information: A randomized-controlled experiment. *Health Communication*, *28*(3), 286–293. doi:10.1080/10410236.2012.683387.

Fröhlich, R. (2008). Political public relations: Research on its success and its influence on German media coverage. In A. Zerfaß, B. v. Ruler, & K. Sriramesh (Eds.), *Public relations research. European and international perspectives and innovations* (pp. 193–204). Wiesbaden: VS.

Fröhlich, R., & Rüdiger, B. (2004). Determinierungsforschung zwischen PR-"Erfolg" und PR-"Einfluss". Zum Potenzial des Framing-Ansatzes für die Untersuchung der Weiterverarbeitung von Polit-PR durch den Journalismus [Determination research between PR "Success" and PR "Influence". The potential of the framing approach for investigating the processing of political PR by journalism]. In J. Raupp & J. Klewes (Eds.), *Quo vadis Public Relations? Auf dem Weg zum Kommunikationsmanagement: Bestandsaufnahme und Entwicklungen [Quo vadis public relations? On the path toward communication management: appraisal and developments]* (pp. 125–141). Wiesbaden: VS.

Fyfe, G., & Law, J. (1988). *Picturing power: Visual depiction and social relations*. London: Routledge.

Gallup. (2014). State of the states. Retrieved from www.gallup.com/poll/125066/State-States.aspx.

Gamson, W. A. (1989). News as framing: Comment on Graber. *American Behavioral Scientist*, *33*(2), 157–161.

Gamson, W. A., Croteau, D., Hoynes, W., & Sasson, T. (1992). Media images and the social construction of reality. *Annual Review of Sociology*, *18*(1992), 373–393.

Gamson, W. A., & Lasch, K. E. (1983). The political culture of social welfare policy. In S. E. Spiro & E. Yuchtman-Yaar (Eds.), *Evaluating the welfare state. Social and political perspectives* (pp. 397–415). New York: Academic Press.

Gamson, W. A., & Modigliani, A. (1987). The changing culture of affirmative action. In R. G. Braungart & M. M. Braungart (Eds.), *Research in political sociology* (Vol. 3, pp. 137–177). Greenwitch, CT: JAI Press.

Gamson, W. A., & Modigliani, A. (1989). Media discourse and public opinion on nuclear power. A constructionist approach. *American Journal of Sociology*, *95*(1), 1–37.

Gandy, O. H. (1982). *Beyond agenda setting: Information subsidies and public policy*. Norwood, NJ: Ablex.

Gandy, O. H. (2001). Epilogue-framing at the horizon: A retrospective assessment. In S. D. Reese, O. H. Gandy, & A. E. Grant (Eds.), *Framing public life: Perspectives on media and our understanding of the social world* (pp. 355–378). Mahwah, NJ: Lawrence Erlbaum.

Gans, H. J. (1980). *Deciding what's news. A study of CBS evening news, NBC nightly news, newsweek and time*. New York: Vintage.

Gans, H. J. (2003). *Democracy and the news*. New York: Oxford University Press.

Garcia, M. R., & Stark, P. (1991). *Eyes on the news*. St. Petersburg, FL: Poynter Institute.

Garner, G. (2007). Photography and society in the 20th century. In M. R. Peres (Ed.), *The focal encyclopedia of photography. Digital imaging, theory and applications, history, and science* (4th ed., pp. 187–198). Boston, MA: Focal Press.

Gausset, Q., Mogensen, H. O., Yameogo, W. M. E., Berthé, A., & Konaté, B. (2012). The ambivalence of stigma and the double-edged sword of HIV/AIDS intervention in Burkina Faso. *Social Science & Medicine*, *74*(7), 1037–1044. doi:10.1016/j.socscimed.2011.11.044.

Gazzaniga, M. S. (1992). *Nature's mind: The biological roots of thinking, emotions, sexuality, language and intelligence*. Harmondsworth: Penguin.

Gazzaniga, M. S. (1998). *The mind's past*. Berkeley: University of California Press.

Geise, S., & Baden, C. (2015). Putting the image back into the frame: Modeling the linkage between visual communication and frame-processing theory. *Communication Theory*, *25*(1), 46–69. doi:10.1111/comt.12048.

Geise, S., Lobinger, K., & Brantner, C. (2013). Fractured paradigm? Theorien, Konzepte und Methoden der visuellen Framingforschung: Ergebnisse einer systematischen Literaturschau [Fractured paradigm? Theories, concepts and methods of visual framing research: Results from a systematic literature review]. In S. Geise & K. Lobinger (Eds.), *Visual framing. Chance und Herausforderung der Visuellen Kommunikationsforschung* (pp. 42–76). Cologne: von Halem.

Gerbner, G., Gross, L., Morgan, M., & Signorielli, N. (1994). Growing up with television: The cultivation perspectives. In J. Bryant & D. Zillmann (Eds.), *Perspectives on media effects* (2nd ed., pp. 17–48). Hillsdale, NJ: L. Erlbaum Associates.

Gibson, R., & Zillmann, D. (2000). Reading between the photographs. The influence of incidental pictorial information on issue perception. *Journalism & Mass Communication Quarterly*, *77*(2), 355–366.

Gilman, S. L. (1988). *Disease and representation: Images of illness from madness to AIDS*. Ithaca, NY: Cornell University Press.

Gilman, S. L. (1995). *Health and illness: Images of difference*. London: Reaktion Books.

Glick, M. H. (2011). Of sodomy and cannibalism: Dehumanisation, embodiment and the rhetorics of same-sex and cross-species contagion. *Gender & History*, *23*(2), 266–282. doi:10.1111/j.1468-0424.2011.01638.x.

Goffman, E. (1963). *Stigma: Notes on the management of spoiled identity*. Englewood Cliffs, NJ: Prentice-Hall.

Goffman, E. (1974). *Frame analysis: An essay on the organization of experience*. Cambridge, MA: Harvard University Press.

Gold, A. L., Cohen, E., & Shumate, M. (2008). Proscriptive models and evidence in antismoking advertising. *Health Communication*, *23*(3), 259–269.

Gordon, I. E. (2004). *Theories of visual perception*. New York: Wiley.

Gould, D. B. (2009). *Moving politics: Emotion and ACT UP's fight against AIDS*. Chicago, IL: University of Chicago Press.

Grabe, M. E. (1996). The SABC's coverage of the 1987 and 1989 elections: The matter of visual bias. *Journal of Broadcasting & Electronic Media*, *40*(1), 1–27.

Grabe, M. E., & Bucy, E. P. (2009). *Image bite politics: News and the visual framing of elections*. Oxford: Oxford University Press.

Grabe, M. E., Lang, A., & Zhao, X. (2003). News content and form: Implications for memory and audience evaluations. *Communication Research*, *30*(4), 387–413. doi:10.1177/0093650203253368.

Graber, D. A. (1976). *Verbal behavior and politics*. Urbana, IL: University of Illinois Press.

Graber, D. A. (1980). *Mass media and American politics*. Washington, DC: Congressional Quarterly Press.

Graber, D. A. (1986). Mass media and political images in elections. *Research in Micropolitics*, *1*(1), 127–160.

Graber, D. A. (1987). Television news without pictures? *Critical Studies in Mass Communication*, *4*(1), 74–78. doi:10.1080/15295038709360115.

Graber, D. A. (1988). *Processing the news: How people tame the information tide* (2nd ed.). New York: Longman.

Graber, D. A. (1990). Seeing is remembering: How visuals contribute to learning from television news. *Journal of Communication*, *40*(3), 134–155.

Graber, D. A. (2001). *Processing politics: Learning from television in the Internet age*. Chicago, IL: University of Chicago Press.

Graber, D. A., & Holyk, G. G. (2012). Civic knowledge and audiovisual learning. In H. A. Semetko & M. Scammell (Eds.), *The sage handbook of political communication* (pp. 153–164). Thousand Oaks, CA: Sage.

Gramsci, A. (1971). *Selections from the prison notebooks*. London: Lawrence and Wishart.

Green, K. E., & Schroeder, D. H. (1990). Psychometric quality of the verbalizer-visualizer questionnaire as a measure of cognitive style. *Psychological Reports*, *66*(3), 939–945.

Griffin, M. (2004). Picturing America's "War on Terrorism" in Afghanistan and Iraq: Photographic motifs as news frames. *Journalism*, *5*(4), 381–402.

Griffin, R. J., & Dunwoody, S. (1995). Impacts of information subsidies and community structure on local press coverage of environmental contamination. *Journalism & Mass Communication Quarterly*, 72, 271–284.

Grimes, T. (1991). Mild auditory-visual dissonance in television news may exceed viewer attentional capacity. *Human Communication Research*, *18*(2), 268–298.

Grimes, T., & Drechsel, R. (1996). Word-picture juxtaposition, schemata, and defamation in television news. *Journalism & Mass Communication Quarterly*, *73*(1), 169–180.

Grittmann, E. (2013). Visual frames-framing visuals. Zum Zusammenhang von Diskurs, Frame und Bild in den Medien am Beispiel des Klimawandeldiskurses [Visual frames-framing visuals. On the relationship between discourse, frame and image in the media with reference to the climate change discourse]. In S. Geise & K. Lobinger (Eds.), *Visual Framing. Chance und Herausforderung der Visuellen Kommunikationsforschung* (pp. 95–116). Cologne: von Halem.

Gross, L. (1991). Out of the mainstream: Sexual minorities and the mass media. *Journal of Homosexuality*, *21*(1–2), 19–46.

Grover, J. Z. (1992). Visible lesions: Images of PWA in America. In J. Miller (Ed.), *Fluid exchanges* (pp. 23–51). Toronto, Canada: Toronto University Press.

Grunig, J. E. (2007). Journalism and public relations. In B. Merkel, S. Russ-Mohl, & G. Zavaritt (Eds.), *A complicated, antagonistic and symbiotic affair: Journalism, public relations and their struggle for public attention* (pp. 101–114). Lugano: Giampiero Gasagrande.

Gunter, B. (2015). *The cognitive impact of television news: Production attributes and information reception*. London: Palgrave Macmillan.

Habermas, J. (1989). *The structural transformation of the public sphere: An inquiry into a category of bourgeois society*. Cambridge, MA: MIT Press.

Hagen, L. M. (1993). Opportune witnesses: An analysis of balance in the selection of sources and arguments in the leading German newspapers' coverage of the census issue. *European Journal of Communication*, *8*(3), 317–343. doi: 10.1177/0267323193008003004.

Hair, J., Black, W., Babin, B., Anderson, R., & Tatham, R. (2006). *Multivariate data analysis*. Trenton, NJ: Pearson Education.

Halawa, M. (2008). *Wie sind Bilder möglich? Argumente für eine semiotische Fundierung des Bildbegriffs [How are Images Possible? Arguments for a semiotic foundation of the image concept]*. Cologne: von Halem.

Hall, S. (1997). *Representation. Cultural representations and signifying practices*. Thousand Oaks, CA: Sage.

Hallahan, K. (1999). Seven models of framing: Implications for public relations. *Journal of Public Relations Research*, *11*(3), 205–242.

Hallahan, K. (2008). Strategic framing. In W. Donsbach (Ed.), *The international encyclopedia of communication*. Blackwell Reference Online: Blackwell Publishing. Retrieved from www.communicationencyclopedia.com/subscriber/tocnode?id=g9781405131995_chunk_g978140513199524_ss112-1. doi:10.1111/b.9781405131995.2008.x.

Hallahan, K. (2015). Strategic framing. In W. Donsbach (Ed.), *The concise encyclopedia of communication* (pp. 600). Malden, MA: Wiley.

Hallet, M. A., & Cannella, D. (1994). Gatekeeping through media format: Strategies of voice for the HIV-positive via human interest news formats and organizations. *Journal of Homosexuality*, *26*(4), 111–134.

Hamilton, J. (2004). *All the news that's fit to sell: How the market transforms information into news*. Princeton, NJ: Princeton University Press.

Hammond, E. (1997). Seeing AIDS: Race, gender, and representation. In N. Goldstein & J. L. Manlowe (Eds.), *The gender politics of HIV/AIDS in women* (pp. 113–116). New York: New York University Press.

Hänggli, R. (2012). Key factors in frame building: How strategic political actors shape news media coverage. *American Behavioral Scientist*, *56*(3), 300–317.

Hänggli, R., & Kriesi, H. (2010). Political framing strategies and their impact on media framing in a swiss direct-democratic campaign. *Political Communication*, *27*(2), 141–157. doi:10.1080/10584600903501484.

Hänggli, R., & Kriesi, H. (2012). Frame construction and frame promotion (Strategic Framing Choices). *American Behavioral Scientist*, *56*(3), 260–278. doi:10.1177/0002764211426325.

Hariman, R., & Lucaites, J. L. (2007). *No caption needed: Iconic photographs, public culture and liberal democracy*. Chicago, IL: University of Chicago Press.

Hastall, M. R., & Knobloch-Westerwick, S. (2012). Severity, efficacy, and evidence type as determinants of health message exposure. *Health Communication*, *28*(4), 378–388. doi:10.1080/10410236.2012.690175.

Hayes, A. F., & Krippendorff, K. (2007). Answering the call for a standard reliability measure for coding data. *Communication Methods and Measures*, *1*(1), 77–89.

Hazelton, M. (1997). Reporting mental health: A discourse analysis of mental health-related news in two Australian newspapers. *Australian & New Zealand Journal of Mental Health Nursing*, *6*(2), 73–89.

Herek, G. M. (1999). AIDS and stigma. *American Behavioral Scientist*, *42*(7), 1106–1116.

Herman, E., & Chomsky, N. (2002). *Manufacturing consent: The political economy of the mass media*. New York: Random House.

Hertog, J. K., Finnegan, J. R., & Kahn, E. (1994). Media coverage of AIDS, cancer, and sexually transmitted diseases: A test of the public arenas model. *Journalism Quarterly*, *71*(2), 291–304.

Hertog, J. K., & McLeod, D. (2001). A multiperspectival approach to framing analysis: A field guide. In S. D. Reese, O. H. Gandy, & A. Grant (Eds.), *Framing public life: Perspectives on media and our understanding of the social world* (pp. 139–161). Mahwah, NJ: Lawrence Erlbaum.

Hickethier, K. (2002). Medien-Aufmerksamkeit. Zur Einführung [Media-attention. An introduction]. In K. Hickethier & J. K. Bleicher (Eds.), *Aufmerksamkeit, Medien und Ökonomie* (pp. 5–13). Hamburg: LIT.

Highleyman, L., & Shepard, B. (2015). Moral reform movements in postwar America. In I. Ness (Ed.), *Encyclopedia of American social movements* (pp. 845–858). New York: Routledge.

Hodes, R. (2007). HIV/AIDS in south African documentary film, c. 1990–2000. *Journal of Southern African Studies*, *33*(1), 153–171.

Hoffman-Goetz, L., Friedman, D., & Clarke, J. N. (2005). HIV/AIDS risk factors as portrayed in mass media targeting first nations, metis, and inuit peoples of Canada. *Journal of Health Communication*, *10*, 145–162.

Hofmann, W. (2008). Die Demokratie der Bilder. Die Risiken und Chancen der audiovisuellen Demokratie [The democracy of images. The risks and rewards of audiovisual democracy]. In A. Brodocz, M. Llanque, & G. S. Schaa (Eds.), *Bedrohungen der Demokratie* (pp. 270–286). Wiesbaden: VS.

Holmqvist, K., Holsanova, J., Barthelson, M., & Lundqvist, D. (2003). Reading or scanning? A study of newspaper and net paper reading. In J. Hyönä, R. Radach, & H. Deubel (Eds.), *The mind's eye. cognitive and applied aspects of eye movement research* (pp. 657–670). Amsterdam: North-Holland.

Holody, K. (2009). *Framing public discourse on physician-assisted suicide: Analysis of newspaper coverage and death with dignity press releases*. Paper presented at the Annual Meeting of the International Communication Association, Chicago, IL.

Holsanova, J., Rahm, H., & Holmqvist, K. (2006). Entry points and reading paths on newspaper spreads: Comparing a semiotic analysis with eye-tracking measurements. *Visual Communication*, *5*(1), 65–93.

Hong, H. (2012). The effects of human interest framing in television news coverage of medical advances. *Health Communication*, *28*(5), 1–9. doi:10.1080/10410236.2012.693013.

Hornig-Priest, S., & Talbert, J. (1994). Mass media and the ultimate technological fix: Newspaper coverage of biotechnology. *Southwestern Mass Communication Journal*, *10*(1), 76–85.

Houts, P. S., Doak, C. C., Doak, L. G., & Loscalzo, M. J. (2006). The role of pictures in improving health communication: A review of research on attention, comprehension, recall, and adherence. *Patient Education and Counseling*, *61*(2), 173–190.

Howe, A. (2006). Crime photography. In L. Warren (Ed.), *Encyclopedia of twentieth-century photography* (Vol. I, pp. 344–346). London: Routledge.

Huang, Y., & Fahmy, S. (2011). *Symbols of nationalism or symbols of repression? The visual framing of the 2008 olympic torch relay in U.S. & Chinese dailies*. Paper presented at the Annual Meeting of the International Communication Association (ICA), Boston, MA.

Hughes, J. (2012). Editor's introduction: SAGE visual methods. In J. Hughes (Ed.), *Sage visual methods* (Vol. I: Principles, Issues, Debates and Controversies in Visual Research, pp. xxi–xlv). Thousand Oaks, CA: Sage.

Hull, K., Smith, L. R., & Schmittel, A. (2015). Form or function? An examination of ESPN magazine's "Body Issue". *Visual Communication Quarterly*, *22*(2), 106–117. doi:10.1080/15551393.2015.1042159.

Hüppauf, B., & Weingart, P. (2009). *Frosch und Frankenstein. Bilder als Medium der Popularisierung von Wissenschaft [Frog and Frankenstein. Images as a medium for the popularization of science]*. Bielefeld: transcript.

Ihlen, Ø., Figenschou, T. U., & Larsen, A. G. (2015). Behind the framing scenes: Challenges and opportunities for NGOs and authorities framing irregular immigration. *American Behavioral Scientist*, *59*(7), 822–838. doi:10.1177/0002764215573254.

Ihlen, Ø., & Nitz, M. (2008). Framing contests in environmental disputes: Paying attention to media and cultural master frames. *International Journal of Strategic Communication*, *2*(1), 1–18.

Janis, I. L., & Fadner, R. (1949). Coefficients of imbalance. In H. Laswell, N. Leites, & Associates (Eds.), *Language of politics*. South Norwalk, CT: George W. Stewart.

Jewitt, C. (2008). Visual representation. In W. Donsbach (Ed.), *The international encyclopedia of communication*. Blackwell Reference Online: Blackwell Publishing. Retrieved from www.communicationencyclopedia.com/subscriber/tocnode?id=g9781405131995_chunk_g978140513199527_ss19-1.

Jewitt, C., & Oyama, R. (2012). Visual meaning: A social semiotic approach. In J. Hughes (Ed.), *Sage visual methods* (Vol. III: Interpretation and Classification, pp. 151–176). Thousand Oaks, CA: Sage.

Joffe, H. (2008). The power of visual material: Persuasion, emotion and identification. *Diogenes*, *55*(1), 84–93. doi:10.1177/0392192107087919.

Johnson-Cartee, K. S. (2004). *News narratives and news framing: Constructing political reality*. Lanham, MD: Rowman and Littlefield.

Jones, R. H. (1997). Marketing the damaged self: The construction of identity in advertisements directed towards people with HIV/AIDS. *Journal of Sociolinguistics*, *1*(3), 393–418.

Juhasz, A. (1990). The contained threat: Women in mainstream AIDS documentary. *Journal of Sex Research*, *27*(1), 25–46.

Juhasz, A. (1993). Knowing AIDS through the televised science documentary. In C. Squire (Ed.), *Women and AIDS: Psychological perspectives* (pp. 150–164). Thousand Oaks, CA: Sage.

Kaniss, P. C. (1991). *Making local news*. Chicago, IL: University of Chicago Press.

Kanwisher, N., McDermott, J., & Chun, M. M. (1997). The fusiform face area: A module in human extrastriate cortext specialized for face perception. *Journal of Neuroscience*, *17*(11), 4302–4311.

Karpf, A. (1988). *Doctoring the media*. London: Routledge.

Kastenbaum, R. J. (2015). *Death, society, and human experience* (11th ed.). London: Routledge.

Kay, A. C., & Eibach, R. P. (2012). The ideological toolbox: Ideologies as tools of motivated social cognition. In S. Fiske & C. N. Macrae (Eds.), *The sage handbook of social cognition* (pp. 495–515). Thousand Oaks, CA: Sage.

Kepplinger, H. M. (1982). Visual biases in television campaign coverage. *Communication Research*, *9*(3), 432–446.

Khamis, S., & Mahmoud, A. E.-B. A. H. (2013). Facebooking the Egyptian elections: Framing the 2012 presidential race. *Journal of Arab & Muslim Media Research*, *6*(2/3), 133–155. doi:10.1386/jammr.6.2-3.133_1.

Khoury, J. (1997). *Implicit propositions in advertising messages: Legal and regulatory aspects*. (M.A. thesis), University of Pennsylvania.

Kilian, E. (2014). Claiming space: Transgender visibility in the arts. In C. Zabus & D. Coad (Eds.), *Transgender Experience. Place, Ethnicity, and Visibility* (pp. 85–100). New York: Routledge.

Kim, S.-H., Besley, J. C., Oh, S.-H., & Kim, S. Y. (2014). Talking about biofuel in the news. *Journalism Studies*, *15*(2), 218–234. doi:10.1080/1461670X.2013.809193.

Kim, S. T., & Weaver, D. H. (2003). Reporting on globalization. A comparative analysis of sourcing patterns in five countries' newspapers. *Gazette*, *65*(2), 121–144. doi:10.1177/0016549203065002002.

King, C., & Lester, P. M. (2005). Photographic coverage during the Persian Gulf and Iraqi wars in three U.S. newspapers. *Journalism & Mass Communication Quarterly*, *82*(3), 623–637. doi:10.1177/107769900508200309.

Kinsella, J. (1989). *Covering the Plague: AIDS and the American Media*. New Brunswick, NJ: Rutgers University Press.

Kiousis, S., Laskin, A., & Kim, J. Y. (2009). *Congressional agenda-building: Examining the influence of congressional communications from the speaker of the house*. Paper presented at the Annual Meeting of the International Communication Association, Chicago, IL.

Kiousis, S., Mitrook, M., Xu, W., & Seltzer, T. (2006). First-and second-level agenda-building and agenda-setting effects: exploring the linkages among candidate news releases, media coverage, and public opinion during the 2002 Florida gubernatorial election. *Journal of Public Relations Research*, *18*(3), 265–285.

Kitch, C. (2009). Tears and trauma in the news. In B. Zelizer (Ed.), *The changing faces of journalism: Tabloidization, technology and truthiness* (pp. 29–39). New York: Routledge.

Kitzinger, J. (1991). Judging by appearances. *Journal of Community & Applied Social Psychology*, *1*(2), 155–163.

Kitzinger, J. (1993). Understanding AIDS: Researching audience perceptions of acquired immune deficiency syndrome. In J. Eldridge (Ed.), *Getting the message* (pp. 271–304). London: Routledge.

Kitzinger, J. (1995). The face of AIDS. In I. Marková & R. M. Farr (Eds.), *Representations of health, illness and handicap* (pp. 49–66). Amsterdam: Harwood.

Klausner, J. D., Kim, A., & Kent, C. (2002). Are HIV drug advertisements contributing to increases in risk behavior among men in San Francisco, 2001? *AIDS*, *16*(17), 2349–2350. doi:10.1097/00002030-200211220-00021.

Kline, K. N. (2014). Media and health, critical analysis of. In T. L. Thompson (Ed.), *Encyclopedia of health communication* (pp. 805–809). Thousand Oaks, CA: Sage.

Knoblauch, H. (2002). Die Gesellschaftliche Konstruktion von Körper und Geschlecht. Oder: Was die Soziologie des Körpers von den Transsexuellen lernen kann [The social construction of body and gender. Or: What can the sociology of the body learn from transsexuals]. In K. Hahn & M. Meuser (Eds.), *Körperrepräsentationen. Die Ordnung des Sozialen und der Körper* (pp. 117–135). Constance: UVK.

Knobloch, S., Hastall, M., Zillmann, D., & Callison, C. (2003). Imagery effects on the selective reading of internet newsmagazines: A cross-cultural examination. *Communication Research*, *30*(1), 3–29.

Knobloch-Westerwick, S., & Sarge, M. A. (2015). Impacts of exemplification and efficacy as characteristics of an online weight-loss message on selective exposure and subsequent weight-loss behavior. *Communication Research*, *42*(4), 547–568. doi:10.1177/0093650213478440.

Kobayashi, S. (1986). Theoretical issues concerning superiority of pictures over words and sentences in memory. *Perceptual and Motor Skills*, *63*(2), 783–792.

Kosicki, G. M., & Pan, Z. (1997). *Defining boundaries and actors in the framing of public discourse*. Paper presented at the Framing in the New Media Landscape Conference, Columbia, SC.

Kress, G. (2010). *Multimodality: A social semiotic approach to contemporary communication*. New York: Routledge.

Kress, G., & van Leeuwen, T. (1996). *Reading images: The grammar of visual design*. New York: Routledge.

Kress, G., & van Leeuwen, T. (1998). Front pages: (The critical) Analysis of newspaper layout. In A. Bell & P. Garrett (Eds.), *Approaches to media discourse* (pp. 186–219). Oxford: Blackwell.

Krippendorff, K. H. (2013). *Content analysis: An introduction to its methodologies*. Thousand Oaks, CA: Sage.

Krishnan, S. P., Durrah, T., & Winkler, K. (1997). Coverage of AIDS in popular African American magazines. *Health Communication*, *9*(3), 273–288.

Kroeber-Riel, W. (1996). *Bildkommunikation. Imagerystrategien für die Werbung [Communication through images. Imagery strategies for advertising]*. Munich: Vahlen.

Küpper, N. (1990). Recording of visual reading activity. Research into newspaper reading behaviour. Retrieved from www.editorial-design.com/leseforschung/Eyetrackstudy.pdf.

Lang, A. (1995). Defining audio/video redundancy from a limited-capacity information processing perspective. *Communication Research*, *22*(1), 86–115.

Lang, A. (2000). The limited capacity model of mediated message processing. *Journal of Communication*, *50*(1), 46–70.

Lang, G. E., & Lang, K. (1981). Watergate: An exploration of the agenda-building process. In C. C. Wilhoit & H. d. Bock (Eds.), *Mass communication review yearbook* (Vol. 2, pp. 447–468). Thousand Oaks, CA: Sage.

Lassiter, G. D., Geers, A. L., Munhall, P. J., Ploutz-Snyder, R. J., & Breitenbecher, D. L. (2002). Illusory causation: why it occurs. *Psychological Science*, *13*(4), 299–305. doi:10.1111/j.0956-7976.2002.x.

Lawrence, R. G. (2010). Researching political news framing: Established ground and new horizons. In P. D'Angelo & J. A. Kuypers (Eds.), *Doing news framing analysis: Empirical and theoretical perspectives* (pp. 265–285). New York: Routledge.

Lazard, A., & Atkinson, L. (2015). Putting environmental infographics center stage: The role of visuals at the elaboration likelihood model's critical point of persuasion. *Science Communication*, *37*(1), 6–33. doi:10.1177/1075547014555997.

Lazarus, R. S. (1998). *Fifty years of the research and theory of R. S. lazarus: An analysis of historical and perennial issues.* Mahwah, NJ: Lawrence Erlbaum.

Lee, S. T. (2014). Predictors of H1N1 influenza pandemic news coverage: Explicating the relationships between framing and news release selection. *International Journal of Strategic Communication*, *8*(4), 294–310. doi:10.1080/1553118X.2014.913596.

Lee, S. T., & Basnyat, I. (2012). From press release to news: Mapping the framing of the 2009 H1N1 A influenza pandemic. *Health Communication*, *28*(2), 119–132. doi:10.1080/10410236.2012.658550.

Lee, S., & Cappella, J. N. (2013). Distraction effects of smoking cues in antismoking messages: Examining resource allocation to message processing as a function of smoking cues and argument strength. *Media Psychology*, *16*(2), 154–176. doi:10.1080/15213269.2012.755454.

Lengauer, G., & Höller, I. (2013). Generic frame building in the 2008 Austrian elections. *Public Relations Review*, *39*(4), 303–314. doi:10.1016/j.pubrev.2013.07.010.

Len-Ríos, M. E., Hinnant, A., Sun-A, P., Cameron, G. T., Frisby, C. M., & Youngah, L. (2009). Health news agenda building: Journalists' perceptions of the role of public relations. *Journalism & Mass Communication Quarterly*, *86*(2), 315–331.

Levy, I., Hasson, U., & Malach, R. (2004). One picture is worth at least a million neurons. *Current Biology*, *14*(11), 996–1001.

Lewis, J., & Jhally, S. (1998). The struggle over media literacy. *Journal of Communication*, *48*(1), 109–120.

Liebler, C., & Bendix, J. (1996). Old-growth forests on network news: News sources and the framing of an environmental controversy. *Journalism & Mass Communication Quarterly*, *73*(1), 53–65.

Liu, Z. (2005). Reading behavior in the digital environment: Changes in reading behavior over the past ten years. *Journal of Documentation*, *61*(6), 700.

Lobinger, K. (2012). *Visuelle Kommunikationsforschung. Medienbilder als Herausforderung für die Kommunikations-und Medienwissenschaft [Visual communication research. Media images as a challenge for communication and media studies]*. Wiesbaden: SpringerVS.

Lobinger, K., & Geise, S. (2013). "Does the frame remain the same?" Visual Framing und Multimodalität als theoretische und methodische Herausforderung der Visuellen Kommunikationsforschung ["Does the frame remain the same?" Visual framing and multimodality as theoretical and methodological challenges of visual communication research]. In S. Geise & K. Lobinger (Eds.), *Visual Framing. Chance und Herausforderung der Visuellen Kommunikationsforschung [Visual framing. Opportunity and challenge for visual communication research]* (pp. 332–357). Cologne: von Halem.

Lundell, Å. K. (2010). The fragility of visuals: How politicians manage their mediated visibility in the press. *Journal of Language & Politics*, *9*(2), 219–236.
Lupton, D. (1994a). *Medicine as culture: Illness, disease and culture in western societies*. Thousand Oaks, CA: Sage.
Lupton, D. (1994b). *Moral threats and dangerous desires*. London: Routledge.
Lupton, D. (1994c). Toward the development of a critical health communication praxis. *Health Communication*, *6*(1), 55–67.
Lupton, D. (1999). Archetypes of infection: People with HIV/AIDS in the Australian press in the mid 1990s. *Sociology of Health & Illness*, *21*(1), 37–53.
Lupton, D. (2000). The social construction of medicine and the body. In G. I. Albrecht, R. Fitzpatrick, & S. C. Scrimshaw (Eds.), *The handbook of social studies in health and medicine* (pp. 50–63). Thousand Oaks, CA: Sage.
Lutz, C. A., & Collins, J. (1993). *Reading national geographic*. Chicago, IL: University of Chicago Press.
Maat, H. P., & de Jong, C. (2013). How newspaper journalists reframe product press release information. *Journalism*, *14*(3), 348–371. doi:10.1177/1464884912448914.
Machin, D., & Niblock, S. (2006). *News production: Theory and practice*. New York: Routledge.
Macken-Horarik, M. (2003). A telling symbiosis in the discourse of hatred: Multimodal news texts about the "Children Overboard" affair. *Australian Review of Applied Linguistics*, *26*(2), 1–16.
Maddux, J. E., & Lopez, S. L. (2015). Deconstructing the illness ideology and constructing and ideology of human strengths and potential in clinical psychology. In S. Joseph (Ed.), *Positive psychology in practice: Promoting human flourishing in work, health, education and everyday life* (2nd ed., pp. 411–428). Hoboken, NJ: John Wiley & Sons.
Martinec, R., & Salway, A. (2005). A system for image-text relations in new (and old) media. *Visual Communication*, *4*(3), 337–371.
Mathers, C. D., & Loncar, D. (2006). Projections of global mortality and burden of disease from 2002 to 2030. *PLoS Medicine*, *3*(11), 2011–2030.
Matthes, J. (2007). *Framing-Effekte. Zum Einfluss der Politikberichterstattung auf die Einstellung der Rezipienten [Framing effects. On the influence of political news on the attitudes of the recipients]*. Munich: Reinhard Fischer.
Matthes, J. (2009). What's in a frame? A content analysis of media framing studies in the world's leading communication journals, 1990–2005. *Journalism & Mass Communication Quarterly*, *86*(2), 349–367.
Matthes, J., & Kohring, M. (2008). The content analysis of media frames: Toward improving reliability and validity. *Journal of Communication*, *58*(2), 258–279.
Mayer, R. E. (1997). Multimedia learning: Are we asking the right questions? *Educational Psychologist*, *32*(1), 1–19.
McAllister, M. P. (1992). AIDS, medicalization, and the news media. In T. Edgar, M. A. Fitzpatrick, & V. S. Freimuth (Eds.), *AIDS: A communication perspective* (pp. 195–221). Hillsdale, NJ: Erlbaum.
McBride, D. M., & Dosher, B. A. (2002). A comparison of conscious and automatic memory processes for picture and word stimuli: A process dissociation analysis. *Consciousness and Cognition*, *11*(3), 423–460.
McCoy, T. S. (1993). *Voices of difference: Studies in critical philosophy and mass communication*. Cresskill, NJ: Hampton.

McCullin, D. (2004). *Life interrupted: HIV/AIDS in Africa*. London: Christian Aid.

McLellan, M., & Steele, B. (2001). Photography and the vulnerable. *The American Editor*, *26*(August), 34.

McLemore, D. M. (2015). Institutional isomorphism and the community structure approach in visual framing of the Trayvon Martin shooting. *Journalism Practice*, *9*(5), 721–740. doi:10.1080/17512786.2014.988993.

McNair, B. (1998). *The sociology of journalism*. London: Arnold.

McWhirter, J. E., & Hoffman-Goetz, L. (2014). A systematic review of visual image theory, assessment, and use in skin cancer and tanning research. *Journal of Health Communication*, *19*(6), 738–757. doi:10.1080/10810730.2013.837562.

Mebane, F., Temin, S., & Parvanta, C. F. (2003). Communicating anthrax in 2001: Comparison of CDC information and print media accounts. *Journal of Health Communication*, *8*(Suppl. 1), 50–82; discussion 148–151.

Mellese, M. A., & Müller, M. G. (2012). Mapping text–visual frames of sub-Saharan Africa in the news: A comparison of online news reports from Al Jazeera and british broadcasting corporation websites. *Communication, Culture & Critique*, *5*(2), 191–229. doi:10.1111/j.1753-9137.2012.01123.x.

Mendelson, A. L., & Thorson, E. (2004). How verbalizers and visualizers process the newspaper environment. *Journal of Communication*, *54*(3), 474–491.

Messaris, P. (1994). *Visual "Literacy": Image, mind, and reality*. Boulder, CO: Westview Press.

Messaris, P. (1997). *Visual persuasion: The role of images in advertising*. Thousand Oaks, CA: Sage.

Messaris, P. (1998). Visual aspects of media literacy. *Journal of Communication*, *48*(1), 70–80.

Messaris, P. (2003). Visual communication: Theory and research. *Journal of Communication*, *53*(3), 551–556.

Messaris, P., & Abraham, L. (2001). The role of images in framing news stories. In S. D. Reese, O. H. Gandy, & A. E. Grant (Eds.), *Framing public life: Perspectives on media and our understanding of the social world* (pp. 215–226). Mahwah, NJ: Lawrence Erlbaum.

Mignault, A., & Chaudhuri, A. (2003). The many faces of a neutral face: Head tilt and perception of dominance and emotion. *Journal of Nonverbal Behavior*, *27*(2), 111–132. doi:10.1023/A:1023914509763.

Mitchell, W. J. T. (1994). *Picture theory: Essays on verbal and visual representation*. Chicago, IL: University of Chicago Press.

Mitchell, W. J. T. (2005). There are no visual media. *Journal of Visual Culture*, *4*(2), 257–266.

Mitchell, A. (2014). State of the news media 2014. Overview. Retrieved from www.journalism.org/2014/03/26/state-of-the-news-media-2014-overview/.

Mondragón, D., Kirkman-Life, B., & Schneller, E. S. (1991). Hostility to people with AIDS: Risk perception and demographic factors. *Social Science & Medicine*, *32*(10), 1137–1142. doi:10.1016/0277-9536(91)90090-Y.

Montgomery, K. C. (1990). Promoting health through entertainment television. In C. Atkin & L. Wallack (Eds.), *Man, communication and public health* (pp. 114–128). Thousand Oaks, CA: Sage.

Moriarty, S. E. (1987). A content analysis of visuals used in print media advertising. *Journalism Quarterly*, *64*(2), 550–554.

Moriarty, S. E., & Popovich, M. N. (1991). Newsmagazines visuals and the 1988 presidential election. *Journalism Quarterly*, *68*(3), 371–380.

Moriarty, S. E., & Show, D. (1995). An antiseptic war: Were news magazines' images of the Gulf War too soft? *Visual Communication Quarterly*, *2*(2), 4–8.

Müller, M. G. (2003). *Grundlagen der Visuellen Kommunikation. Theorieansätze und Analysemethoden [A primer for visual communication. Theoretical approaches and analytical methods]*. Constance: UTB.

Müller, M. G. (2007). What is visual communication? Past and future of an emerging field of communication research. *Studies in Communication Sciences*, *7*(2), 7–34.

Müller, M. G. (2013). »You cannot unsee a picture!« Der Visual-Framing-Ansatz in Theorie und Empirie [»You cannot unsee a picture!« The visual framing approach in theory and empirical research]. In S. Geise & K. Lobinger (Eds.), *Visual Framing Perspektiven und Herausforderungen der Visuellen Kommunikationsforschung* (pp. 19–41). Cologne: von Halem.

Muturi, N., & An, S. (2010). HIV/AIDS stigma and religiosity among African American women. *Journal of Health Communication*, *15*(4), 388–401.

Ndiaye, K. (2014). Stigmatization, consequences of. In T. L. Thompson (Ed.), *Encyclopedia of health communication* (pp. 1335–1336). Thousand Oaks, CA: Sage.

Nelkin, D. (1987). *Selling science: How the press covers science and technology*. New York: Freeman.

Nelkin, D. (1991). AIDS and the news media. *The Milbank Quarterly*, *69*(2), 293–307.

Nelson, D. L., & Castano, D. (1984). Mental Representations for Pictures and Words: Same or Different? *American Journal of Psychology*, *97*(1), 1–15.

Nelson, T. E., & Willey, E. (2001). Issue frames that strike a value balance: A political psychology perspective. In S. D. Reese, O. H. Gandy, & A. E. Grant (Eds.), *Framing public life: Perspectives on media and our understanding of the social world* (pp. 245–266). Mahwah, NJ: Lawrence Erlbaum Associates.

Netter, T. W. (1992). The media and AIDS: A global perspective. In J. Sepulveda, H. Fineberg, & J. Mann (Eds.), *AIDS: Prevention through education: A world view* (pp. 241–253). New York: Oxford University Press.

Newell, A. (1990). *Unified theories of cognition*. Cambridge, MA: Harvard University Press.

Newman, J. (2014). *Utopia and terror in contemporary American fiction*. New York: Routledge.

Newport, F. (2013). Mississippi maintains hold as most religious U.S. state. Retrieved from www.gallup.com/poll/160415/mississippi-maintains-hold-religious-state.aspx.

Newton, J. H. (2001). *The burden of visual truth: The role of photojournalism in mediating reality*. Mahwah, NJ: Erlbaum.

Niederdeppe, J., Davis, K. C., Farrelly, M. C., & Yarsevich, J. (2007). Stylistic features, need for sensation, and confirmed recall of national smoking prevention advertisements. *Journal of Communication*, *57*(2), 272–292.

Niederdeppe, J., Shapiro, M. A., & Roh, S. (2014). *Consequences of failure to acknowledge individual responsibility in narratives designed to promote public policies to reduce rates of obesity*. Paper presented at the 64th Annual Meeting of the International Communication Association, Seattle, WA.

Noller, P. (1985). Video primacy-a further look. *Journal of Nonverbal Behavior, 9*(1), 28–47.

Norris, R. L., Bailey, R. L., Bolls, P. D., & Wise, K. R. (2012). Effects of emotional tone and visual complexity on processing health information in prescription drug advertising. *Health Communication, 27*(1), 42–48. doi:10.1080/10410236.2011.567450.

Nucci, M. L., Cuite, C. L., & Hallman, W. K. (2009). When good food goes bad: Television network news and the spinach recall of 2006. *Science Communication, 31*(2), 238–265.

Olesen, T. (2012). Televised media performance for HIV/AIDS sufferers in Africa: Distance reduction and national community in two Danish fundraising shows. *Communication, Culture & Critique, 5*(1), 99–119.

O'Malley, D. A., & Latimer-Cheung, A. E. (2013). Gaining perspective: The effects of message frame on viewer attention to and recall of osteoporosis prevention print advertisements. *Journal of Health Psychology, 18*(11), 1400–1410.

O'Neill, D., & O'Connor, C. (2008). The passive journalist. How sources dominate local news. *Journalism Practice, 2*(3), 487–500. doi:10.1080/17512780802281248.

O'Toole, A. J. (2005). Psychological and neural perspectives on human face recognition. In S. Z. Li & A. K. Jain (Eds.), *Handbook of face recognition*. New York: Springer.

Ott, B. L., & Mack, R. L. (2014). *Critical media studies: An introduction* (2nd ed.). Malden, MA: Wiley.

Paivio, A. (1979). *Imagery and verbal processes*. Hillsdale, NJ: Psychology Press.

Paivio, A. (1986). *Mental representations. A dual coding approach*. Oxford: Oxford University Press.

Paivio, A. (1991). Dual coding theory: Retrospect and current status. *Canadian Journal of Psychology/Revue canadienne de psychologie, 45*(3), 255–287. doi:10.1037/h0084295.

Paivio, A., & Csapo, K. (1973). Picture superiority in free recall: Imagery or dual coding? *Cognitive Psychology, 5*(2), 176–206.

Pan, Z., & Kosicki, G. M. (1993). Framing analysis: An approach to news discourse. *Political Communication, 10*(1), 55–75.

Pan, Z., & Kosicki, G. M. (2001). Framing as a strategic action in public deliberation. In S. D. Reese, O. H. Gandy, & A. E. Grant (Eds.), *Framing public life: Perspectives on media and our understanding of the social world* (pp. 35–65). Mahwah, NJ: Lawrence Erlbaum.

Park, K. (1993). Kimberly bergalis, AIDS, and the plague metaphor. In M. Garber, J. Matlock, & R. Walkowitz (Eds.), *Media spectacles* (pp. 232–253). New York: Routledge.

Parker, A. (2003). *In the blink of an eye: How vision sparked the big bang of evolution*. New York: Perseus.

Parry, K. (2010). A visual framing analysis of British press photography during the 2006 Israel-Lebanon conflict. *Media, War & Conflict, 3*(1), 67–85. doi:10.1177/1750635210353679.

Parry, K. (2011). Images of liberation? Visual framing, humanitarianism and British press photography during the 2003 Iraq invasion. *Media, Culture & Society, 33*(8), 1185–1201. doi:10.1177/0163443711418274.

Patterson, T. E. (1994). *Out of order.* New York: Vintage.

Patterson, A. S. (2014). Societal dynamics, state relations, and international connections: Influences on Ghanaian and Zambian church mobilization in AIDS treatment. In R. van Dijk, H. Dilger, M. Burchardt, & T. Rasing (Eds.), *Religion and AIDS treatment in Africa: Saving souls, prolonging lives* (pp. 197–222). New York: Routledge.

Perrault, E. K., & Silk, K. J. (2014). Testing the effects of the addition of videos to a website promoting environmental breast cancer risk reduction practices: Are videos worth it? *Journal of Applied Communication Research, 42*(1), 20–40. doi:10.1080/00909882.2013.854400.

Petty, R. E., & Cacioppo, J. T. (1984). The elaboration likelihood model of persuasion. *Advances in Consumer Research, 19*, 673–675.

Pfau, M., Haigh, M., Fifrick, A., Holl, D., Tedesco, A., Cope, J., ... Martin, M. (2006). The effect of print news photographs of the casualties of war. *Journalism & Mass Communication Quarterly, 83*(1), 150–168.

Pickle, K., Quinn, S. C., & Brown, J. D. (2002). HIV/AIDS coverage in black newspapers, 1991–1996: Implications for health communication and health education. *Journal of Health Communication, 7*(5), 427–444.

Pieterse, J. M. (1992). *White on black: Images of Africa and blacks in western popular culture.* New Haven, CT: Yale University Press.

Pitts, M., & Jackson, H. (1993). Press coverage of AIDS in Zimbabwe: A five-year review. *AIDS Care, 5*(2), 223–230.

Poindexter, P. M., Heider, D., & McCombs, M. E. (2006). Watchdog or good neighbor? The public's expectations of local news. *Harvard International Journal of Press/Politics, 11*(1), 77–88.

Pollack, E., & Allern, S. (2014). Criticism of the police in the news. *NORDICOM Review, 35*(1), 33–50.

Pollock, J. C. (2007). *Tilted mirrors: Media alignment with political and social change: A community structure approach.* Cresskill, NJ: Hampton Press.

Posner, M. I., Nissen, M. J., & Klein, R. M. (1976). Visual dominance: An information-processing account of its origins and significance. *Psychological Review, 83*(2), 157–171.

Postman, N. (1986). *Amusing ourselves to death: Public discourse in the age of show business.* New York: Penguin.

Potter, G. W., & Kappeler, V. E. (1998). *Constructing crime: Perspectives on making news and social problems.* Long Grove, IL: Waveland Press.

Powell, T. E., Boomgaarden, H. G., De Swert, K., & de Vreese, C. H. (2015). A clearer picture: The contribution of visuals and text to framing effects. *Journal of Communication, 65*(6), 997–1017. doi:10.1111/jcom.12184.

Powers, A., & Andsager, J. L. (1999). How newspapers framed breast implants in the 1990s. *Journalism & Mass Communication Quarterly, 76*(3), 551–564.

Pratt, C. B., Ha, L., & Pratt, C. A. (2002). Setting the public health agenda on major diseases in sub-saharan Africa: African popular magazines and medical journals, 1981–1997. *Journal of Communication, 52*(4), 889–904.

Price, V., & Feldman, L. (2008). News processing and retention. In W. Donsbach (Ed.), *The international encyclopedia of communication.* Blackwell Reference Online: Blackwell Publishing. Retrieved from www.communicationencyclopedia.com/subscriber/tocnode?id=g9781405131995_chunk_g978140513199519_ss26-1.

Price, V., & Tewksbury, D. (1997). News values and public opinion: A theoretical account of media priming and framing. In G. Barnett & F. Boster (Eds.), *Progress in communication sciences* (Vol. 13, pp. 173–212). Greenwich, CT: Ablex.

Princeton Survey Research Associates. (1996, July/August). Covering the epidemic: AIDS in the news media, 1985–1996. *Columbia Journalism Review, 35*(Special supplement).

Quinlan, M. M. (2014). Media depictions: Disability. In T. L. Thompson (Ed.), *Encyclopedia of health communication* (pp. 824–826). Thousand Oaks, CA: Sage.

Raupp, J. (2008). Determination theory in public relations. In W. Donsbach (Ed.), *The international encyclopedia of communication* (pp. 1222–1226). Malden, MA: Blackwell.

Raupp, J. (2014). Social agents and news media as risk amplifiers: A case study on the public debate about the *E. coli* outbreak in Germany 2011. *Health, Risk & Society, 16*(6), 565–579. doi:10.1080/13698575.2014.950203.

Reber, B. H., & Berger, B. K. (2005). Framing analysis of activist rhetoric: How the Sierra Club succeeds or fails at creating salient messages. *Public Relations Review, 31*(2), 185–195.

Reese, S. D. (2007). The framing project: A bridging model for media research revisited. *Journal of Communication, 57*(1), 148–154.

Reese, S. D., Gandy, O. H., & Grant, A. E. (Eds.). (2001). *Framing public life: Perspectives of media and our understanding of the social world.* Mahwah, NJ: Lawrence Erlbaum.

Reich, Z. (2006). The process model of news initiative. Sources lead first, reporters thereafter. *Journalism Studies*, 7(4), 497–514. doi:10.1080/14616700600757928.

Reich, Z. (2009). *Sourcing the News. Key Issues in Journalism.* Cresskill, NJ: Hampton Press.

Reich, Z. (2010). Measuring the impact of PR on published news in increasingly fragmented news environments-A multifaceted approach. *Journalism Studies, 11*(6), 799–816.

Reynolds, A., & Barnett, B. (2003). "America under Attack": CNN's verbal and visual framing of september 11. In S. M. Chermak, F. Y. Bailey, & M. Brown (Eds.), *Media representations of September 11* (pp. 85–102). Santa Barbara, CA: Greenwood Publishing Group.

Riles, J. M., Sangalang, A., Hurley, R. J., & Tewksbury, D. (2015). Framing cancer for online news: Implications for popular perceptions of cancer. *Journal of Communication, 65*(6), 1018–1040. doi:10.1111/jcom.12183.

Rim, H., Lee, B.-G., & Han, J. W. (2009). *The Influence of News Sources on Health News Content: Does Localization Really Matter?* Paper presented at the Annual Meeting of the International Communication Association (ICA), Chicago, IL.

Ritchin, F. (1990). *In our own image. The coming revolution in photography.* New York: Aperture.

Rodriguez, L., & Dimitrova, D. V. (2011). The levels of visual framing. *Journal of Visual Literacy, 30*(1), 48–65.

Rogers, E., Dearing, J., & Chang, S. (1991). AIDS in the 1980s: The agenda-setting process for a public issue. *Journalism Monographs, 126*(1), 1–46.

Roosvall, A. (2016). Religion, globalization and commodification in online world news slideshows: The dis/connection of images and texts. *Social Semiotics*, *26*(1), 76–93. doi:10.1080/10350330.2015.1059581.

Rose, G. (2012). *Visual methodologies. An introduction to the interpretation of visual materials* (3rd ed.). Thousand Oaks, CA: Sage.

Rosenblum, B. (1978). Style as social process. *American Sociological Review*, *43*(3), 422–438.

Rosenblum, K. E., & Travis, T. C. (1996). Constructing categories of difference: Framework essay. In K. E. Rosenblum & T. C. Travis (Eds.), *The meaning of difference: American constructions of race, sex and gender, social class, and sexual orientation* (pp. 1–34). New York: McGraw-Hill.

Ryan, C. (1991). *Prime time activism: Media strategies for grassroots organizing*. Boston, MA: South End Press.

Ryan, C., & Gamson, W. A. (2009). Are frames enough? In J. Goodwin & J. M. Jasper (Eds.), *The social movements reader: Cases and concepts* (pp. 167–174). Chichester: Blackwell.

Sacks, V. (1996). Women and AIDS: An analysis of media misrepresentations. *Social Science & Medicine*, *42*(1), 59–73.

Salwen, M. B. (1995). News of hurricane andrew: The agenda of sources and the sources' agendas. *Journalism & Mass Communication Quarterly*, *72*(4), 826–840. doi:10.1177/107769909507200406.

Scalvini, M. (2010). Glamorizing sick bodies: How commercial advertising has changed the representation of HIV/AIDS. *Social Semiotics*, *20*(3), 219–231.

Scheufele, D. A. (1999). Framing as a theory of media effects. *Journal of Communication*, *49*(1), 103–122.

Scheufele, D. A. (2000). Agenda-setting, priming, and framing revisited: Another look at cognitive effects of political communication. *Mass Communication and Society*, *3*(2), 297–316. doi:10.1207/S15327825MCS0323_07.

Scheufele, B. (2001). Visuelles Medien-Framing und Framing-Effekte. Zur Analyse visueller Kommunikation aus der Framing-Perspektive [Visual media framing and framing effects. For the analysis of visual communication from the framing perspective]. In T. Knieper & M. G. Müller (Eds.), *Kommunikation visuell. Das Bild als Forschungsgegenstand. Grundlagen und Perspektiven [Visual Communication. The picture as a research object. Basics and perspectives]* (pp. 144–158). Cologne: von Halem.

Schiller, H. (1973). *The mind managers*. Boston, MA: Beacon.

Schreier, M. (2012). *Qualitative content analysis in practice*. Thousand Oaks, CA: Sage.

Schudson, M. (1991). The sociology of news production revisited. In J. Curran & M. Gurevitch (Eds.), *Mass media and society* (pp. 141–328). London: Edward Arnold.

Schudson, M. (2003). *The sociology of news*. New York: Norton.

Schudson, M. (2006). The trouble with experts-and why democracies need them. *Theory and Society*, *35*, 491–506.

Schwalbe, C. B. (2006). Remembering our shared past: Visually framing the Iraq war on U.S. news websites. *Journal of Computer-Mediated Communication*, *12*(1), 264–289.

Schwalbe, C. B., Silcock, B. W., & Keith, S. (2008). Visual framing of the early weeks of the U.S.-led invasion of Iraq: Applying the master war narrative to

electronic and print images. *Journal of Broadcasting & Electronic Media, 52*(3), 448–465.
Schwan, S., & Zahn, C. (2006). Der Bildbetrachter als Gegenstand bildwissenschaftlicher Methodik [The image viewer as an object of research in visual studies]. In K. Sachs-Hombach (Ed.), *Bild und Medium. Kunstgeschichtliche und philosophische Grundlagen der interdisziplinären Bildwissenschaft* (pp. 214–232). Cologne: von Halem.
Schwartz, D. (1992). To tell the truth: Codes of objectivity in photojournalism. *Communication, 13*(2), 95–109.
Schwitzer, G. (1992). The magical medical media tour. *Journal of the American Medical Association, 267*(14), 1969–1972.
Semetko, H. A., Blumler, J. G., Gurevitch, M., & Weaver, D. H. (1991). *The formation of campaign agendas: A comparative analysis of party and media roles in recent American and British elections.* Hillsdale, NJ: Lawrence Erlbaum.
Semetko, H. A., & Valkenburg, P. M. (2000). Framing European politics: A content analysis of press and television news. *Journal of Communication, 50*(2), 93–109.
Seo, K., & Shen, F. (2009). *The interactive effects of visual images and message framing on health-related persuasion.* Paper presented at the Annual Meeting of the International Communication Association (ICA), Chicago, IL.
Sharf, B. F., & Vandeford, M. L. (2003). Illness narratives and the social construction of health. In T. L. Thompson, A. Dorsey, K. I. Miller, & R. Parrott (Eds.), *Handbook of health communication* (pp. 9–34). Mahwah, NJ: Lawrence Erlbaum.
Sheafer, T., & Gabay, I. (2009). Mediated public diplomacy: A strategic contest over international agenda building and frame building. *Political Communication, 26*(4), 447–467.
Shoemaker, P. J. (1991). *Gatekeeping.* Thousand Oaks, CA: Sage.
Shoemaker, P. J., & Reese, S. D. (1996). *Mediating the message: Theories of influences on mass media content* (2nd ed.). White Plains, NY: Longman.
Shoemaker, P. J., & Reese, S. D. (2014). *Mediating the message in the 21st century: A media sociology perspective* (3rd ed.). New York: Routledge.
Shook, F. (2000). *Television field production and reporting.* New York: Longman.
Sigal, L. V. (1973). *Reporters and officials: The organization and politics of newsmaking.* Lexington, MA: D. C. Heath.
Sigal, L. V. (1986). Sources make the news. In R. K. Manoff & M. Schudson (Eds.), *Reading the news* (pp. 9–37). New York: Pantheon.
Smith, N. E. (2006). *Stem cell research: Visual framing of the ethical debate in Time and Newsweek.* Paper presented at the Annual Convention of the Association for Education in Journalism and Mass Communication, San Francisco, CA.
Sontag, S. (1989). *AIDS and its metaphors.* London: Penguin.
Sotirovic, M., & McLeod, J. M. (2004). Knowledge as understanding: The information processing approach to political learning. In L. L. Kaid (Ed.), *Handbook of political communication research* (pp. 357–394). Mahwah, NJ: Lawrence Erlbaum Associates.
Southwell, B. G. (2005). Between messages and people: A multilevel model of memory for television content. *Communication Research, 32*(1), 112–140. doi:10.1177/0093650204271401.

Spinetta, C. M. (2014). Ideological hegemony. In T. L. Thompson (Ed.), *Encyclopedia of health communication* (pp. 687–689). Thousand Oaks, CA: Sage.

Stark Adam, P., Edmonds, R., & Quinn, S. (2007). *Eyetracking the news. A study of print and online reading*. St. Petersburg, FL: The Poynter Institute.

Stenfors, I., Morén, J., & Balkenius, C. (2003). Behavioural strategies in web interaction: A view from eye-movement research. In J. Hyönä, R. Radach, & H. Deubel (Eds.), *The mind's eye. Cognitive and applied aspects of eye movement research* (pp. 633–644). Amsterdam: Elsevier.

Stocking, S. H. (1985). Effects of public relations efforts on media visibility of organizations. *Journalism Quarterly*, *62*(2), 358–366.

Strömbäck, J., & Esser, F. (2009). Shaping politics: Mediatization and media Interventionism. In K. Lundby (Ed.), *Mediatization, concepts, changes, consequences* (pp. 205–223). New York: Peter Lang.

Strömbäck, J., Negrine, R., Hopmann, D. N., Jalali, C., Berganza, R., Seeber, G. U. H., ... Maier, M. (2013). Sourcing the news: Comparing source use and media framing of the 2009 European parliamentary elections. *Journal of Political Marketing*, *12*(1), 29–52. doi:10.1080/15377857.2013.752227.

Strömbäck, J., & Nord, L. W. (2006). Do politicians lead the tango?: A study of the relationship between Swedish journalists and their political sources in the context of election campaigns. *European Journal of Communication*, *21*(2), 147–164. doi:10.1177/0267323105064043.

Stryker, J. E. (2008). Health communication and journalism. In W. Donsbach (Ed.), *The international encyclopedia of communication*. Blackwell Reference Online: Blackwell Publishing. Retrieved from www.communicationencyclopedia.com/subscriber/tocnode.html?id=g9781405131995_chunk_g978140513199513_ss12-1. doi:10.1111/b.9781405131995.2008.x.

Sturken, M. (1997). *Tangled memories*. Berkeley: University of California Press.

Swain, K. A. (2005). Approaching the quarter-century mark: AIDS coverage and research decline as infection spreads. *Critical Studies in Media Communication*, *22*(3), 258–262.

Swain, K. A. (2007). Outrage factors and explanations in news coverage of the anthrax attacks. *Journalism & Mass Communication Quarterly*, *84*(2), 335–352.

Swift, A. (2014). Wyoming residents most conservative, D.C. Most Liberal. Retrieved from www.gallup.com/poll/167144/wyoming-residents-conservative-liberal.aspx.

Tagg, J. (1988). *The burden of representation: Essays on photographies and histories*. Basingstoke: Macmillan.

Tankard, J. W. (2001). The empirical approach to the study of media framing. In S. D. Reese, O. H. Gandy, & A. Grant (Eds.), *Framing public life: Perspectives on media and our understanding of the social world* (pp. 95–106). Mahwah, NJ: Lawrence Erlbaum.

Tanner, A. H. (2004). Agenda building, source selection, and health news at local television stations. *Science Communication*, *25*(4), 350–363.

Tanner, A. H., & Friedman, D. B. (2011). Authorship and information sourcing for health news on local TV web sites: An exploratory analysis. *Science Communication*, *33*(1), 3–27. doi:10.1177/1075547010364926.

Tedesco, J. C. (2001). Issue and strategy agenda-setting in the 2000 presidential primaries. *American Behavioral Scientiest*, *44*(12), 2048–2067.

Temoshok, C., Grade, M., & Zich, J. (1988). Public health, the press and AIDS: An analysis of newspaper articles in London and San Francisco. In I. B. Corless & M. Pittman-Lindeman (Eds.), *AIDS: Principles, practices and politics* (reference ed., pp. 535–552). New York: Hemisphere.

Tewksbury, D., Jones, M., Peske, A. R., & Vig, W. (2000). The interaction of news and advocate frames: manipulating audience perceptions of a local policy issue. *Journalism & Mass Communication Quarterly*, *77*(4), 804–830.

The Foundation for AIDS Research (amfAR). (2011). Thirty years of HIV/AIDS: Snapshots of an epidemic. Retrieved from www.amfar.org/thirty-years-of-hiv/aids-snapshots-of-an-epidemic/.

Tiemens, R. K. (1978). Television's portrayal of the 1976 presidential debates: An analysis of visual content. *Communication Monographs*, *45*(4), 362–370.

Trautman, T. C. (2004). Concerns about crime and local television news. *Communication Research Reports*, *21*(3), 310–315.

Treichler, P. A. (1988a). AIDS, gender, and biomedical discourse. In E. Fee & D. M. Fox (Eds.), *AIDS: The burdens of history* (pp. 190–266). Berkeley: University of California Press.

Treichler, P. A. (1988b). AIDS, homophobia, and biomedical discourse: An epidemic of signification. In D. Crimp (Ed.), *AIDS, cultural analysis, cultural activism*. Cambridge, MA: MIT.

Treichler, P. A. (1999). *How to have theory in an apidemic: Cultural chronicles of AIDS*. Durham, NC: Duke Press.

Tuchman, G. (1978). *Making news. A study in the construction of reality*. New York: Free Press.

Turk, J. V. (1985). Information subsidies and influence. *Public Relations Review*, *11*(3), 10–25.

Turner, M. M., Skubisz, C., Pandya, S. P., Silverman, M., & Austin, L. L. (2014). Predicting visual attention to nutrition information on food products: The influence of motivation and ability. *Journal of Health Communication*, *19*(9), 1017–1029. doi:10.1080/10810730.2013.864726.

Turow, J., & Coe, L. (1993). Curing television's ills: The portrayal of health care. In B. C. Thornton & G. L. Kreps (Eds.), *Perspectives on health communication* (pp. 130–145). Prospect Heights, IL: Waveland.

United States Census Bureau. (2014). Urban and Rural. Retrieved from www2.census.gov/geo/docs/reference/ua/PctUrbanRural_State.xls.

Unz, D. C. (2007). Emotional Framing-Wie audiovisuelle Medien die emotionale Verarbeitung beeinflussen [Emotional Framing – How audiovisual media affects emotional processing]. In A. Bartsch, J. Eder, & K. Fahlenbrach (Eds.), *Audiovisuelle Emotionen. Emotionsdarstellung und Emotionsvermittlung durch audiovisuelle Medienangebote [Audiovisual emotions. The presentation and conveyance of emotions through audiovisual media]* (pp. 238–255). Cologne: von Halem.

Valentino, N. A. (1999). Crime news and the priming of racial attitudes during evaluations of the president. *Public Opinion Quarterly*, *63*(3), 293–320. doi:10.1086/297722.

Van Gorp, B. (2005). Where is the Frame? Victims and Intruders in the Belgian Press Coverage of the Asylum Issue. *European Journal of Communication*, *20*(4), 484–507.

Van Gorp, B. (2007). The constructionist approach to framing: Bringing culture back in. *Journal of Communication*, *57*(1), 60–78.

Van Gorp, B. (2010). Strategies to take subjectivity out of framing analysis. In P. D'Angelo & J. A. Kuypers (Eds.), *Doing news framing analysis: Empirical and theoretical perspectives* (pp. 84–109). New York: Routledge.

Van Gorp, B., Vettehen, P. H., & Beentjes, J. W. J. (2009). Challenging the frame in the news. The role of issue involvement, attitude, and competing frames. *Journal of Media Psychology*, *21*(4), 161–170.

Van Hoof, A., Takens, J., & Oegema, D. (2010). *Poor framing in television news: Redundancy between audio and visual modalities in political news*. Paper presented at the Annual Meeting of the International Communication Association (ICA), Singapore, Singapore.

Van Leeuwen, T., & Jewitt, C. (2001). *Handbook of visual analysis*. Thousand Oaks, CA: Sage.

Viswanath, K. (2006). Public communications and its role in reducing and eliminating health disparities. In G. E. Thomson, F. Mitchell, & M. B. Williams (Eds.), *Examining the health disparities research plan of the National Institutes of Health: Unfinished business* (pp. 215–253). Washington, DC: Institute of Medicine.

Vobič, I., & Tomanić Trivundža, I. (2015). The tyranny of the empty frame. *Journalism Practice*, *9*(4), 502–519. doi:10.1080/17512786.2015.1030137.

Waisbord, S. (2015). My vision for the journal of communication. *Journal of Communication*, *65*(4), 585–588. doi:10.1111/jcom.12169.

Wanta, W., & Roark, V. (1994). Response to photographs. *Visual Communication Quarterly*, *1*(2), 12–13.

Washington, H. (2006). *Medical apartheid: The dark history of medical experimentation on black Americans from colonial times to the present*. New York: Doubleday.

Waters, E. A., McQueen, A., & Cameron, L. D. (2013). Perceived risk and its relationship to health-related decisions and behavior. In L. R. Martin & M. R. DiMatteo (Eds.), *The oxford handbook of health communication, behavior change, and treatment adherence* (pp. 193–213). Oxford: Oxford University Press.

Watney, S. (1988). AIDS, "Moral Panic" Theory and homophobia. In P. Aggleton & H. Homans (Eds.), *Social aspects of AIDS* (pp. 52–64). Lewes: Falmer Press.

Watney, S. (1990a). Missionary position: AIDS, "Africa, " and Race. In R. Ferguson, M. Gever, T. T. Minh-ha, & C. West (Eds.), *Out there: Marginalization and contemporary cultures* (pp. 89–103). New York: The New Museum of Contemporary Art.

Watney, S. (1990b). Photography and AIDS. In C. Squiers (Ed.), *The critical image: Essays on contemporary photography* (pp. 173–192). Seattle, WA: Publishers Press.

Watts, L. (1993). *Coverage of polio and AIDS*. (PhD thesis), Scripps School of Journalism, Athens, OH.

Weaver, D. H., & Elliott, S. N. (1986). Who sets the agenda for the media? A study of local agenda building. *Journalism Quarterly*, *62*, 87–94.

Weeks, J. (1988). Love in a cold climate. In P. Aggleton & H. Homans (Eds.), *Social aspects of AIDS* (pp. 10–19). Lewes: Falmer Press.

Wehmeier, S. (2008). Intereffication approach in public relations. In W. Donsbach (Ed.), *The international encyclopedia of communication*. Blackwell Reference Online: Blackwell Publishing. Retrieved from www.communicationencyclopedia.com/subscriber/tocnode.html?id=g9781405131995_yr2015_chunk_g978140513199514_ss53-1.

Weissman, P. L. (2014). *Where does news about prescription drugs come from? Exploring how organizations built and framed the national news media agenda for hormone therapy from 1995 to 2011*. (PhD thesis), University of Maryland, College Park, MD.

Wellings, K. (1988). Perception of risk-media treatment of AIDS. In P. Aggleton & H. Homans (Eds.), *Social aspects of AIDS* (pp. 83–105). London: Falmer Press.

Wessler, H., Wozniak, A., Hofer, L., & Lück, J. (2016). Global multimodal news frames on climate change: A comparison of five democracies around the world. *The International Journal of Press/Politics*, *21*(4), 423–445. doi:10.1177/1940161216661848.

Whitaker, R. (2013). Medical reporting. In B. Turner & R. Orange (Eds.), *Specialist journalism* (pp. 147–159). New York: Routledge.

Wießner, P. (2004). Aids und Werbung [AIDS and advertising]. In AIDS Forum DAH (Ed.), *AIDS im Wandel der Zeiten [AIDS in the course of time]* (Vol. 47, pp. 47–54). Berlin: Deutsche AIDS-Hilfe e.V.

Williams, K., & Miller, D. (1995). AIDS news and news cultures. In J. Downing, A. Mohammadi, & A. Sreberny-Mohammadi (Eds.), *Questioning the media* (2nd ed., pp. 413–427). Thousand Oaks, CA: Sage.

Wise, D., & Brewer, P. R. (2010). Competing frames for a public health issue and their effects on public opinion. *Mass Communication and Society*, *13*(4), 435–457.

Wolf, H. (2008). The tears of photography. *Grey Room*, *29*(Winter), 66–89.

Wolf, R., & Grotta, G. L. (1985). Images: A question of readership. *Newspaper Research Journal*, *6*(2), 30–36.

Woollacott, J. (1982). Messages and meanings. In M. Gurevitch, T. Bennett, J. Curran, & J. Woollacott (Eds.), *Culture, society and the media* (pp. 91–111). New York: Routledge.

Yan, C. (2015). Persuading people to eat less junk food: A cognitive resource match between attitudinal ambivalence and health message framing. *Health Communication*, *30*(3), 251–260. doi:10.1080/10410236.2013.842525.

Ye, Y., & Ward, K. E. (2010). The depiction of illness and related matters in two top-ranked primetime network medical dramas in the United States: A content analysis. *Journal of Health Communication*, *15*(5), 555–570. doi:10.1080/10810730.2010.492564.

Zhou, Y., & Moy, P. (2007). Parsing framing processes: The interplay between online public opinion and media coverage. *Journal of Communication*, *57*(1), 79–98.

Zillmann, D. (2006). Exemplification effects in the promotion of safety and health. *Journal of Communication*, *56*(s1), S221-S237. doi:10.1111/j.1460-2466.2006.00291.x.

Zillmann, D., & Brosius, H.-B. (2000). *Exemplification in communication: The influence of case reports on the perception of issues*. Mahwah, NJ: Lawrence Erlbaum.
Zillmann, D., Gibson, R., & Sargent, S. L. (1999). Effects of photographs in news-magazine reports on issue perception. *Media Psychology*, *1*(3), 207–228.
Zillmann, D., Knobloch, S., & Yu, H.-s. (2001). Effects of photographs on the selective reading of news reports. *Media Psychology*, *3*(4), 301–324.
Zoller, H. M. (2014). Critical approaches. In T. L. Thompson (Ed.), *Encyclopedia of health communication* (pp. 270–273). Thousand Oaks, CA: Sage.

Index